ESSENTIAL
FORENSIC
PATHOLOGY

Core Studies and Exercises

ESSENTIAL FORENSIC PATHOLOGY

Core Studies and Exercises

Gilbert Edward Corrigan

CRC Press
Taylor & Francis Group
Boca Raton London New York

CRC Press is an imprint of the
Taylor & Francis Group, an **informa** business

CRC Press
Taylor & Francis Group
6000 Broken Sound Parkway NW, Suite 300
Boca Raton, FL 33487-2742

First issued in paperback 2020

ISBN-13: 978-1-4398-7666-4 (hbk)
ISBN-13: 978-0-367-77855-2 (pbk)

Library of Congress Cataloging-in-Publication Data

Corrigan, Gilbert Edward.
  Essentials of forensic pathology : core studies and exercises / Gilbert Edward Corrigan.
    p. ; cm.
  Includes bibliographical references and index.
  ISBN 978-1-4398-7666-4 (hardback : alk. paper)
  I. Title.
  [DNLM: 1. Forensic Pathology--education--Problems and Exercises. W 618.2]

614'.1--dc23   2011050404

Visit the Taylor & Francis Web site at
http://www.taylorandfrancis.com

and the CRC Press Web site at
http://www.crcpress.com

Contents

Section IV
DEDICATION

The Author

Gilbert Edward Corrigan was born on May 3, 1929, in Cleveland, Ohio, and grew up during the Great Depression and World War II. His father was a trial lawyer and his mother a journalist. He studied biology at Adelbert College of Western Reserve University majoring in evolution and genetics (under Amos Hersh, PhD). Corrigan studied evolution at Notre Dame University (under Edward O. Dodson, PhD) and moved to The Ohio State University where he studied human genetics (under Madge Macklin, PhD) and anatomy (under Linden Forest Edwards, PhD). He taught anatomy at Wayne State University in Detroit, Michigan, and graduated from medical school with honors in psychiatry. Following his internship at Harper Hospital in Detroit, he qualified in pathology by training at The Ohio State University (under E. Von Hamm, MD), Boston Children's Hospital (Sidney Farber, MD), and the Maryland Medical Examiner's Office (Russell Fisher, MD). Corrigan has practiced pathology over 40 years at 10 institutions. He is board certified in anatomical and forensic pathology. He plays and composes on the saxophone and is an active member of the St. Louis Track Club. He also promotes the Missouri Academy of Science (moacadsci.org).

Introduction

I

Introduction: Coaching Objectives in Medical Education

1

In the 1970s, coincidental with the advent of the personal computer, there arrived a time of consideration of educational technique in U.S. medical education. There was a voiced appeal for new medical schools, which gained support. At that time, a change was made so that all medical schools and all medical students would be exposed to a similar education method and content. A national standard was contemplated and was opened to any medical school graduate in the world whose education met measured standards. The change from written essay questions was founded on the utility of multiple choice questions, which allowed automated grading and methods of comparison of tested schools and classes. The subjectivity of the written test was gone. The content of the doctor of medicine (MD) degree would be overviewed and critiqued as allowed by this new testing method. The essay test, so revered for its required literary skills and unprompted answers, died a quick and sudden death in undergraduate and graduate medical education.

In the newly formed Group for Research in Pathology Education (GRIPE), there was a strong move for gathering and compilation of the testing data and curricular materials used in pathology courses led by the GRIPE president Thomas Kent, MD. A concern arose that students and teachers should know, exactly and precisely, the objectives for each course Printed objectives allowed concise comparisons of courses. All of the course materials were stated in each medical school curricular catalog. This was a driving and powerful educational mandate and was stimulated by the increasing involvement of the medical schools with federal governmental sponsoring of medical education. At this time, twenty new medical schools were opened under federal support.

Objectives are classified as *robust* when they show measurable learning outcomes in the domains of knowledge, skills, and behaviors. Usually, objectives are divided in their use and application into two groups: basic science objectives or clinical science objectives. Generally, the better the written objectives, the better is the school. Remember, one person (like myself) can sit down and write an entire book of objectives … which would take an entire team of writers to present in textbook detail. Voila.

The writing of objectives was easy for me, as I had years of experience writing and grading the broadest of test materials—the written essay examination. Today the essay exam is a testing method restricted to the assessment of students in legal and graduate studies. As a teacher my essay questions were fashioned to start a student in the right direction with a quiz item, which allowed the student's complete definition of the stated problem and yet had some limitations to its boundaries. A good essay exam will reward the savant and give him or her unlimited space to achieve a complete demonstration of mastery of the topic area approached. Students who were less prepared would find the test a fair venue for the exposure of what they knew and understood. The same goals are shared in the structure of the course objectives presented here.

My pedagogical skills were honed in the large anatomy department of The Ohio State University where I received my PhD degree. I became a friend of the large classroom. As a lab instructor of things anatomical, I went from a junior assistant instructor to an assistant instructor in five years, worked with dental and nursing students, and taught all of the medical school anatomy courses several times. My degree was as much a teaching degree as a research degree. In those days a professor at my alma mater Ohio State was ranked by the number of graduate and undergraduate students he or she taught and not by the amount of his research grants.

Later my educational background was strengthened by an active membership in the Group of Research in Pathology Education (GRIPE) and work in concepts of medical and pathology education on a national level. At meetings of the International Association of Medical School Educators (IAMSE) my focus was on the entire medical school curriculum. (As an aside, one of my students became the president of Harvard Medical School and one the president of Johns Hopkins Medical. Could it be that the Midwestern work ethic thrives on the East Coast?)

Objectives in Forensic Pathology Training

The objectives compiled in this book should meet the highest of standards and present each student with a framework on which complete demonstration of understanding the subject matter at hand can develop. No key subjects are neglected or omitted. These objectives are meant to define the topic at hand just as the strokes of an artist's brush define the painting. The mastery of these objectives parallels the mastery of forensic pathology as an academic subject.

Personally, I recommend that those starting out do a rapid survey of the contents of this study of forensic pathology and then spend one day or night a week on each section with a periodic summative review of all that is covered until all sections have been conquered. After mastery of the individual sections, one is prompted by the teaching ethic of our academic discipline to create another special section by oneself and extend its contents to other students in the most available method at hand, such as on the Internet, as a meeting bulletin board topic, as a separate written discourse, or an oral presentation. In other words, try writing your own objectives for what you are learning.

I envisioned an academic utility for this work and took these objectives and fashioned them to fit a full academic course of a 16-week semester with three meetings a week. This allows for an easily arranged course outline with 46 separate topic areas of the academic subject of forensic pathology. Two periods are designated as test days: an accumulative test at the half-way point, covers the first half of the course materials, and a summative test at the end of the course, which covers the entire course.

Beginning physicians may not know how to limit their intellectual curiosity and restrict their studies to forensic pathology and its related topics. Be sure to stick to the topic of forensic pathology. It is tempting to develop a parallel interest in the law; however, the law and forensic pathology have different dimensions, responsibilities, and goals. Some can achieve both law and medical degrees; however, the responsibilities for knowledge and achievement in both fields are only managed well by a few savants. Most students are either scientists or lawyers. However, the American Academy of Forensic Sciences has specialization sections in related fields, including criminalistics, pathology/biology, and psychiatry/behavioral science. Forensic pathology is a young science and is still maturing and developing. Membership in the American Academy of Forensic Sciences will acquaint you with the people responsible for the rapid and extensive expansion that is taking place in all of the forensic sciences. The modern forensic pathologist is challenged by the massive increase in scientific detail and must rely on his knowledge of computer skills and informatics to maintain a leadership position on the expanding margins of the forensics sciences. For physicians, a solid base in the basic medical sciences is necessary.

The literature of forensic pathology and legal medicine is rich and universal. The use of the secondhand book service from Amazon cannot be denied as a ready and primary site for scholars. I have had great success on the Internet using Amazon as a book search.

A Program in Forensic Pathology

II

A directory of pathology training programs is published yearly by the Intersociety Committee on Pathology Information (ICPI), 4733 Bethesda Avenue, Suite 700, Bethesda, MD 20814 (phone: 301-656-2942). Certification is by the American Board of Pathology, P.O. Box 25915, Tampa, FL 33622-5915 (phone: 813-286-2444). The board also sells a set of questions.

The Forensic Pathology Residency Program with Rotations

2

A forensic pathology residency program includes the following rotations:

Admission interview
Autopsy (morgue) rotation
Toxicology rotation
Anthropology rotation
Homicide rotation (scenes, police services, courtroom)
Crime lab rotation
Neuropathology rotation (to include psychiatric relationships)
Forensic and surgical pathology rotation (slide review) with immuno-histochemistry
Research rotation (visiting conventions and presenting at meetings)
Public health and environmental health rotation
Military forensic pathology rotation
Forensic biology and entomology rotation
Transportation pathology rotation
Forensic pathology office management rotation (visiting other training sites and forensic offices)
Forensic odontology rotation (when not a part of the autopsy or first rotation)

Most forensic pathology programs omit significant attention to digital and multimedia services, engineering sciences, jurisprudence, and questioned documents all of which are sections within the American Academy of Forensic Sciences (AAFS). Note that for a period of time (less than ten years) the forensic path residency was two years in duration. I would find no difficulty in providing a two-year curriculum for forensic pathology, however, the realities of forensic practice allow constant learning to be a by-product of the methodology.

That is each case is a learning experience. Also inherent in forensic pathology is the responsibility to understand the inventiveness of the criminal mind, and the challenge to the forensic pathologist to always be ready to expose and explain crimes that have never been studied before. This is especially true with death from poisoning.

The Residency Admission Interview

It is important that there be an eye-to-eye meeting of the resident candidate with the chief forensic pathologist who will guide the education at a personal level. His or her associate pathologists, the office and laboratory staff, administrator, and any available classmates may be included. A plan for the training is agreed to by all and understood by all. A calendar is agreed to, and the beginning and end of the training is defined and dated. While all of the details of the rotations may not be finalized, at least a blocking out of the assignments is made. Items to be agreed upon include weekend and vacation rotations, computer privileges and information system responsibilities, sick leave and hospitalization, family matters for married residents, hospital staff privileges, and the details of the work contract with the fiduciary agent.

This is an opportunity to bridge moral, religious, social, and ethical concerns that might become major problems if not evaluated and solved prior to service. Items include prior arrests and convictions, classification as a sex offender or mental health deviant, incomplete educational training, failures in certification testing, problems in citizenship, uncompleted military obligations, and inadequate verification of training and graduation. An open review should be made of any of the student's ongoing legal obligations and a plan of fulfillment established. The dominance of the chief pathologist in the formal decisions of the office is defined. Finally financial support of the student for the period of study should be assured. A confirmatory letter of appointment shall be sent.

Plans for an exit interview may be made at this time and a concern for the placement of the resident may be shown.

Section Outline for Resident Rotation in Forensic Pathology

Ten fields apply to each rotation:

1. Name of rotation
2. Faculty monitor/manager
   a. Qualifications
3. Place and facility
4. Forensic workload
5. Evidentiary product
6. Current methodology
7. Necessary skills
8. Laboratory equipment
9. Recording equipment
10. Safety discipline

The Forensic Pathology Residency

The prime objective of the forensic pathology residency is to ensure the residents' capacity to perform a good and complete forensic autopsy. Although most residents have previous autopsy experience, that is not necessarily the circumstance. An evaluation of each resident and his or her capabilities is necessary. Experience with the usual (classic) types of forensic autopsies to be encountered in a typical community practice is emphasized. The autopsy is repeated in a standard fashion and practiced in an intense manner enabling the distinctive acts of a forensic autopsy to become second nature and habitual, for example, the precise dissection of the coronary artery system. Training has always been localized in morgues with a substantial load of homicide cases, as homicides are a critical ingredient in the forensic case mix. Indeed, the majority of the rotations through the anatomical autopsy services were focused on homicide, with experiences extending from the scene investigation to the final courtroom appearance under oath.

In 2010 there were 25 training sites in the United States listed by the American Board of Pathology. Generally, their training topics include autopsy pathology, toxicology, criminalistics and crime lab experience, anthropology, homicide team analysis, forensic biology, neuropathology, forensic and surgical pathology, histology, research, environmental pathology, forensic biology, and entomology. Implicit in most programs are the recognition of military, transportation, public health, legal (testimonial), and environmental aspects of forensic pathology. There are no apparent remnants of previous exercises in a two-year forensic path residency.

Following are some small items of practical utility for new residents:

1. Use Google and Yahoo search engines to keep informed of forensic matters. They will save you all of the news items on forensics and deliver them to you for free. I use four headings: coroner, medical examiner, forensic autopsy, and forensic pathologist. I either print or download the stories. After several years you will get a rhythm for what reporters report; it has its limitations.
2. Do search the Web and before you start downloading a bunch of stuff, look around as much is duplicated. Search forensic pathology, medical examiner, and topics that interest you.
3. Cruising through the Amazon book catalog is a cool way to learn the literature. Before buying, check out the book from the nearest library.
4. Do get a camera and become a shutterbug; learn how to use the printer on your computer to put out a good picture. We all should know Photoshop software. You should be able to match the police sergeant at the scene.

5. Skilled use of a cell phone camera is great for forensic team communication. Be sure all are informed, equipped, and know how to use the gear.
6. You should spend the year perfecting your autopsy techniques, which includes fine dissections, and special organ dissections of the brain, heart, lungs, liver, kidneys, guts, and so forth. Make a mental list of your needed (wanted) technical skills and do them one at a time.
7. Learn your computer software, both that of your institution and that of your personal ownership. Master all Microsoft Office programs.
8. Do not hesitate to understand the local and regional politics but understand your presence as an educated professional may upset some politicians. A legal education is now at your disposal with excellent legal schooling available over the Internet. Note that other equivalently supportive degrees (like an MBA or a master's in ethics, computer science, or public health) are also available on the Internet and are well respected. The private practice of forensic pathology was an unusual start for most pathologists because of the lack of finances and experience. However, things have changed and with the proper training and connections you can start right out. Forensic pathology can be a successful entrepreneurial business enterprise if your family and wallet will allow it.
9. The coroner system has one thing over the medical examiner system in that the coroner system is directly involved with the psychiatric problems of the community through its ability to impound people. Forensic pathology is closely related to clinical psychiatry through the legal control of emergency hospitalizations of psychotic patients. Most medical examiner systems are only loosely involved with the community mental health problems.
10. The job of the resident in his or her education is to secure the MD license, pass the forensic boards, secure the appropriate state licenses, take care of the business of employment as needed, maintain a hospital position as needed, have a plan to pay off any school debts, attend to professional creativity (writing, inventions, services) through associations, and keep smiling.

The forensic pathology training rotations are as follows.

Autopsy Rotation

The autopsy rotation will include a mixture of cases by age, sex, occupation, social level, manner of death, toxicological and physical mechanisms, political importance, and difficulty of dissection. The major case groups are homicides, suicides, overdoses, work accidents, sudden natural death without medical records, motor vehicle accidents, drownings, abortions, accidental shootings, and geriatric deaths. The critical educational ingredient for the beginner in working these cases is the tutelage of an experienced healthy observant senior pathologist who is capable of provoking interest in seemingly mundane events and things, and who can integrate or summate the multiple disease events and pathophysiological factors into a complete understandable scientific explanation (diagnosis). The intensity of forensic practice requires a layering of this expertise in the forensic pathology staff. It takes more than one. Resident assessment methods include written essay exams, multiple choice exams, monitored interviews of scene personnel and families, software use including statistical programs, database management, and forensic identification software. Postautopsy review of the pathological changes found at autopsy is a critical teaching method.

The autopsy experience of each resident assigned to a case is derived from different separate activities learned as a progression in detail. This includes monitoring the informational data from the death scene; management of the flow of the scientific information from the corpse and its adjuvant studies such as trace evidence and immune histochemistry; complete corpse dissection as designated by the institutional protocol; setting up special studies and organ conferences; histological processing of the tissues; the ordering, cataloging, and recording of the essential nonautopsy diagnostic studies, such as x-rays; providing a report on the diagnosis and meaning of the tissue and cytology examinations; and conferring with the attending case pathologist on the final diagnosis and final report. A final diagnosis is formulated and used in the monitoring of the autopsy surgeon's experience.

The containers with histology and saved representative tissues are consecutively numbered, labeled, sealed, stored, and recorded.

Each case is signed out under the preceptorship of one of the staff pathologists; both the resident and the preceptor sign out the case. Problems are referred to the chief pathologist.

The resident learns what to take away from each completed autopsy dissection. This will include the written dissection notes and organ weight sheet. These handheld papers show the ballistic measurements for each entry and exit wound (note: these are not or may not be finalized until the final protocol is typed or dictated), and any preserved special dissection specimens (e.g., eyeballs with hemorrhage from child abuse cases). A note on the x-rays should be part of the case file and maintained with the records. The x-rays are usually stored in a separate file in an area with the other anatomical specimens (i.e., cytology, histology, and special study specimens).

Although residents may enter the program with varying quantities and varieties of experience, at the end of this intensive year of studying the submitted cases, a general sufficiency of experience is present and has been recorded as a person record. The program director and the resident pathologist assume the responsibility for the quality of the program. Attention is paid to the differences in both pediatric and geriatric pathology.

Historically there was no attempt in most programs to teach or develop entrepreneurial skills in student pathologists to promote the establishment of new offices or to extend the role of forensic pathology in the medical community. This has been an individualized responsibility not taught in the residency training and presumed to be available to those who wanted to learn the political and management skills necessary for program development either in a medical examiner's office or a coroner's office. A journal devoted to the management of public death facilities appeared for the first time in 2010: *Forensic Pathology: Policy and Management.*

1. Name of rotation: Forensic autopsy, forensic pathology proper.
2. Faculty monitor/manager: Supervising pathologist with diener staff (diener is a morgue worker; the word is German for "servant").
   a. Qualifications: A board-certified forensic pathologist with several years of experience, good health, appropriate teaching disposition, and defined term of office.

      The diener staff should be adequate in strength and number, managed by written protocol with annual reviews, schooled in morgue hygiene and waste disposal, clean by habit, and well supported by an attentive professional computerized administration.

      Residents are a part of the morgue administration.
3. Place and facility: Each dissection facility needs adequate and clean workspace with clean dissection areas, safe floors and lighting, hygienic cleaning routines, adequate space for storage and equipment, appropriate lighting, safe and comfortable airflow, and responsible management with written and recorded protocols including yearly management reviews. A complete radiological service is provided with the x-ray machine, films and film storage, development chemicals and developing facilities, reading facilities.

   Residents should be active in morgue management and assist in the daily management tasks.
4. Forensic workload: The workload is managed by written protocol reviewed annually with administration.

   Residents should share the workload professionally and also find methods for studying particular case types according to their research protocols and research interests. Outside consultations are given in cases inside and outside the area of responsibility. The model of disease employed is the biopsychosocial model.

5. Evidentiary products: The principal evidentiary product is the written autopsy protocol and the compiled coroner/medical examiner report.

    The compiled report includes the written reports of all of the functionary members of the death investigation team; the medical examiner/coroner defines the report as complete as appointed manager of the case and determiner of the cause of death. Reports and consultations are logged.

6. Current methodology: The current autopsy dissection protocol is unchanged over several centuries (open all body cavities and describe/define the contents). However, new physical methods of body part visualization arise each year and may be used in body analysis according to the evidentiary needs of the case. The radiological examination of the bodies both in the instance of demonstration of gunshot pellets and in evaluation of skeletal trauma and fractures is integral to this training activity. The resident is to provide the complete radiological analysis from placement of the films and the radiological probe to the examination of the images and their diagnosis.

7. Necessary skills: The resident pathologist uses this year of monitored autopsy experience to learn the nuances and fine points of forensic anatomy dissection and histological/cytological visualization. The resident also learns management and storage of radiological equipment and films.

8. Laboratory equipment: A simple dissection room in a funeral home requires improved portable lighting and a strict code of postmortem cleanliness and disposal. A simple concrete block building can be converted to a mortuary provided there is an adequate dissection room with proper aeration and disposal; a refrigerated body storage area; a chemical supply storage area; a shelved tissue storage area; a file room; a prosector's and pathologist's suite with shower, toilet, and changing room; a conference room with communications and computers; a truck and vehicle garage; a secretarial office; an identification area; and a waiting room.

9. Recording equipment: The forensic photography equipment (purchased and managed by the professional photographer who is responsible for the photographic product) will provide case documentation and an opportunity for resident pathologists to learn the important details of forensic photography. Ceiling cameras with continuous recording require authorization, security, regulation, and professional management with authorization/review of the case pathologist.

10. Safety discipline: The discipline of safety in the practice of pathology must be a part of the anatomical rotation as the diagnosis and recognition of infectious disease is a significant public health function of forensic pathology; protection of all health workers is a required part of the practice of forensic pathology. Proper safety practice requires education, statements of principle, drills and practices, routine examinations, and proper record keeping. An appointed safety officer is a key person in this operation when given adequate responsibility and management power.

Toxicology Rotation

1. Name of rotation: Toxicology.
2. Faculty monitor/manager: The director of the toxicology section provides a direct contact for the resident to the large worldwide enterprise of forensic toxicology. The toxicology director knows the members of the forensic and chemical industry toxicology establishment. He or she knows the marketplace of toxicological instrumentation and the grant writing skills necessary to secure modern equipment. The daily analytical functioning of the lab is an important responsibility and is managed according to written procedures with precision and accuracy.

 The fifty or so analytical procedures are all documented and detailed for professional and court review. Since some procedures require overnight processing and "next-day analysis" a timetable and weekly scheduling is necessary. The tox lab is managed in a controlled and careful manner. Duplicate analysis is employed as needed.

 An active part and role in the scientific evidentiary status of current and proposed toxicological practices provide a foundation for discussions on the important elements of modern forensic toxicology. The laboratory director shows a complete mastery of the written protocols on diagnostic technique and quality control in the tox lab.
  a. Qualifications: Keen analytical chemical skills, knowledge of modern computerized automated equipment with management skills, appropriate forensic experience, maintains inspection readiness, capable of consulting with the medical staff. Most have a university doctorate degree. Some may work with residents on a supported toxicological study.
3. Place and facility: The tox lab should be convenient to the training facility and house all of the major functional toxicological analytical instruments; the residents should be comfortably housed and the working areas well lighted and free of obstructions. Room for resident and faculty research is required.

4. Forensic workload: The workload should be manageable and under control. The case mix should be varied and standard automation should be employed where the workload is appropriate.
5. Evidentiary product: The written report is provided in document fashion to all involved parties and the courtroom testimony available as needed by the law. A yearly summary of court appearances is formalized and numerical analysis is used. Reports and consultations are logged.
6. Current methodology: Screening tests for alcohol has retained a role, gas chromatography is applied to the alcohols and other volatiles using known standards, chromatography retains a position, and the gas chromatography combined with the mass spectrophotometer is the major instrument in a varied package of physical detectors. Extensive libraries of analytical information are computerized for identification.
7. Necessary skills: The resident-in-training should be able to do the routine work of the toxicology technical staff. This includes laboratory weighing, pipette calibration, the use of various pipettes (micro-, macro-, automated), stirring, pouring, and mixing, lab notebook management, use of safety equipment and respirators, inflammable storage, fire prevention, and written report skills.
8. Laboratory equipment: A major forensic office has at least a half a million dollars in analytical instrumentation when combined with the computer programming necessary for management of the growing caseload.
9. Recording equipment: Residents should be able to take photographs at all magnifications, understand/use scanning electron microscopes, and provide illustrations of particulate materials with beam scanning.
10. Safety discipline: Safety regulations are reviewed and discussed, and safety drills are enacted throughout the rotation. The role of the safety office is reviewed.

Anthropology Rotation

1. Name of rotation: Forensic anthropology, physical anthropology, anthropology, human forensic anatomy.
2. Faculty monitor/manager: The anthropologist or anatomist under contract by the forensic office to supply anthropological and anatomical services.
   a. Qualifications: A graduate degree in anatomy or anthropology, experience and training in forensic anatomy and/or anthropology, manager of a working forensic unit with diagnostic qualifications.

3. Place and facility: An anatomical amphitheatre with analytical space, microscopic facilities, spot chemical capabilities, trace evidence capability, qualitative and quantitative chemical study, forensic photography with spectroscopy, skeletonization facility, bone and skeleton storage, bone disease analysis as required, tissue storage with freezing capacity, tissue processing with histology equipment, x-ray diagnostic unit, and other analytical instruments.

   A computer network with complete scientific service software and adequate network connections that function in the recording of the daily office work should be open and available to the resident pathologists.

4. Forensic workload: Discovered human and animal parts, discovered skeletons and bodies, problem findings of unknown origin, radiological studies, workup of disasters and disaster scenes, volunteer efforts in adjacent and international scenes, forensic consultations with tissue procurement for forensic purposes.

   The irregular and sporadic nature of body and body part discovery requires an adaptation scheme in the resident work schedule so that the residents may take part in special scenes and body examinations that become special because of the circumstances of their discovery or relationships. This workload should be available to residents when these special opportunities for service and research arise.

5. Evidentiary product: A complete scientific report includes a studied (referenced) and carefully stated anatomical or anthropological diagnosis correlated with the circumstances of the discovery and its forensic meaning; descriptive scientific data; and cataloged photography, scans, and x-ray specimens. Reports and consultations are logged.

6. Current methodology: Gross, microscopic, and molecular biological and chemical studies based on well-referenced, evidence-based analytical scheme analyzed by experienced and certified scientists.

7. Necessary skills: Modern analytical skills with computer resource support; appropriate time allocations and proper space accommodations and housing; supported ethical standards.

8. Laboratory equipment: Microscopes, cameras, x-ray machines and scanners, communications equipment, and modern software for scientific analysis and management.

9. Recording equipment: Photography, video, and radio, with courtroom presentation and enactment capability.

10. Safety discipline: A written and reviewed safety program with active participation and annual review; the proper storage of all explosive and volatile chemicals and objects; an appointed safety officer with management contact; prion disease precautions.

Homicide Rotation (Scenes, Police Services, Courtroom)

The homicide rotation presents a unique opportunity for the residen: to learn the creed and behavior of the modern police homicide unit. The resident is introduced to the homicide unit officially at the morning meeting, is paired with a detective team, and follows the team through several scenes while learning the daily routine of the homicide investigation. The team is followed through the various sectors of the departmental forensic science network and the methods of informational synthesis are learned. A nighttime patrol car shift provides valuable experience.

The detectives are followed to their courtroom appearance and the initial steps of the homicide prosecution are demonstrated. An interview with a prosecuting attorney provides knowledge of the formal legal needs of the state in homicide prosecution.

1. Name of rotation: Homicide case rotation.
2. Faculty monitor/manager: One of the active homicide detective teams working cases that go to the morgue for final analysis.
   a. Qualifications: The detective team should be willing and expository in nature.
3. Place and facility: Police department detective offices.
4. Forensic workload: The resident partakes in homicide scene investigations and works with the assigned detective team. Read all the true crime stories and memoirs of forensic pathologists that you can find, borrow, or buy. Study your local homicide staff and ask questions.
5. Evidentiary product: The homicide detective provides his analysis of his assigned cases to departmental superiors and they provide the evidence to the prosecutor; in the absence of a direct prosecution, relationships are made with other law enforcement agencies to further the evidentiary trail in the case. Reports and consultations are logged.
6. Current methodology: The last decade has seen a proliferation of computer software in all aspects of forensic informatics including morgue, coroner, and medical examiner case logs; individual case management schemes; indexing of cases by geodesic, census, political, tax base, employment, and other factors; and advanced computer search systems based on Java and other computer languages.
7. Necessary skills: Residents passing through this rotation should develop skills in the understanding of the police ethics in homicide investigation, knowledge of the local applicable legal police privileges, knowledge on the closing of cases, and obtaining legal public confessions.
8. Laboratory equipment: The residents on the homicide rotation should have experience with scene and search lighting, trace evidence

collection and equipment, forensic photography, and simple finger-print collection suitable for basic morgue utilization.

9. Recording equipment: Cameras, computers, photo lab software, and sound recording equipment suitable for taping interviews.
10. Safety discipline: Includes the use and management of bulletproof vests and clothing, basic bomb and anthrax protection protocols with practice sessions, attention to the presence of shooters at public aggregations, arson and its various patterns of utilization, driver and passenger safety, dangers of high-speed pursuits, dealing with car-jacking episodes, and gun-safety rules and regulations.

Crime Lab Rotation

The crime lab rotation covers the following criminalistics:

1. DNA
2. Serology
3. Light microscopy
4. Forensic photography
5. Ballistics
6. Trace evidence with infrared/ultraviolet radiation
7. Computer science evidentiary findings
8. Forensic informatics and computer analysis

The crime lab rotation should give the forensic pathology resident an idea of the areas of responsibility covered by the lab, how deep into the specific iden-tification of items the lab will go, the relationship of the technical staff to the instrumentation and the goals of analysis, how they present their materials in court, the relationship of the lab to other police and federal labs, and the use of the lab data in prosecution and case solving.

The connection of the autopsy data and the crime scene data with other forensic science details should be studied and the varying relationships under-stood. Independent study of the various fields of the forensic sciences is neces-sary and attendance at forensic science sales conventions should be promoted.

The residents should spend some time at the bench overseeing the tech-niques and recordkeeping of forensic science practitioners working in the office. Advances in digital methods should be reviewed and the routine for the evaluation of a computer taken into evidence should be experienced.

The collection of the trace evidence from the body in the controlled envi-ronment of the morgue provides manageable and precise evidentiary work. Evidence collection may also be performed at the scene or in the hospital emergency room. The housing of this function at the morgue provides for more sophisticated collection and identification methods. These forensic collection skills may be evaluated in the crime lab rotation. Do review your qualitative chemistry from college.

Neuropathology Rotation (to Include Psychiatric Relationships)

The neuropathology rotation is a very empowering rotation for a pathologist. Following this experience, which builds confidence in anatomical analysis of the cut brain, the resident can conduct his or her own weekly, biweekly, or monthly conference. The brain-cutting conference is a major socialization source of cooperation and problem solving for the scientists, technicians, physicians, and pathologists caring for the living and dead victims of forensic trauma. Selection of cases for further study and publication are made at this conference.

Accommodations for residents with insufficient psychiatric experience can be made and ancillary teaching rounds established.

1. Name of rotation: Neuropathology with brain-cutting conference and psychiatric conferences.
2. Faculty monitor/manager: Staff neuropathologist and associates in neurohistopathology.
   a. Qualifications: Board certified neuropathologist or equivalent experience in traumatic, vascular, and advanced forensic neuropathology.
3. Place and facility: A neuropathology laboratory including a conference room with brain-cutting facilities, a neurohistological laboratory with diagnostic microscopy services, brain storage areas, library, slide storage areas, professional offices and secretarial suite.
4. Forensic workload: Approximately 10 to 20 percent of forensic autopsies are facilitated by neuropathology; many are determined by the neuropathology findings. Following the biopsychosocial medical model in the interpretation of disease, analysis of the psychiatric aspects of each case is established.
5. Evidentiary product: A written report with scientific documentation to include neuropathology specimens with definitive advanced histological and analytical techniques.
6. Current methodology: Brain cutting followed by histology, neurohistology with silver stains, immunohistology, viral studies, meningitis studies, prion and other infectious diseases, pediatric and geriatric analysis, drug overdose and asphyxial deaths. Reports and consultations are logged.
7. Necessary skills: Found in anatomical pathology, pediatric pathology, geriatric pathology, neuropathology, developmental studies, microbiology, and general pathology.

8. Laboratory equipment: Large whole-brain microtome, a complete histology laboratory, x-ray and CAT scan capability, scanners.
9. Recording equipment: Photography, video, and radio, with courtroom presentation and enactment capability.
10. Safety discipline: Includes special precautions in the management of prion infected tissues and the successful management of prion disease tissues. The information management of communitywide viral and bacterial brain diseases is also a critical responsibility.

Forensic and Surgical Pathology Rotation

The forensic histology materials for the week are combined with a surgical pathology rotation with immunohistochemistry and genetic relationships. The unique histology of forensic pathology is completely reviewed on a weekly basis and all of the major disease vectors studied. Generally at least one slide from each case is processed through this conference. Histopathological records are maintained.

The diagnostic skills of the general anatomical pathology are maintained by a well-defined weekly review of fresh surgical cases. At least one hour a week is attached to this duty. Cases of tumors and histologically defined conditions found at forensic autopsy also are presented.

1. Name of rotation: Forensic and surgical pathology with immunohistochemistry on a weekly basis.
2. Faculty monitor/manager: The assigned pathologist with rotational surgical duties.
   a. Qualifications: Board certified in anatomical pathology.
3. Place and facility: A diagnostic teaching multiheaded microscope; a digital microscope with projection capacity.
4. Forensic workload: About 1 to 2 percent of forensic cases relate to precise histopathological identification of diseases and tumors.
5. Evidentiary product: A carefully executed forensic pathology diagnosis is established by the resident. Reports and consultations are logged.
6. Current methodology: Both conventional and digital histopathology slides are reviewed and continuing medical education records maintained.
7. Necessary skills: Tissue identification, cell and tissue analysis with precise evaluation of the mode and manner of disease.
8. Laboratory equipment: Current standard histopathological equipment, both digital and conventional; conventional continuing medical education materials are utilized.
9. Recording equipment: Photography, video, and radio, with courtroom presentation and enactment capability.

10. Safety discipline: Conventional safety equipment with a standard safety program, which is monitored, fully equipped, and evaluated in a timely manner.

Research Rotation

Taxing agencies at all levels have found that the research grant method of fund dispersal allows them more freedom to do what they want to do than any other method of support. Distributing funds through the grant method allows the endowing agency complete control of all of the circumstances of fund distribution. Operational funding through grants is a government-wide method; it has pervaded all of the private elements as well.

The topic of grant writing has become a bona fide academic exercise; courses at all levels are available. Residents should use the research rotation to hone their skills in grant writing. The research rotation provides an opportunity to start research in a topic area or a research methodology that appeals to the resident. It is a good time to start because one is around other pathologists who are doing research in the same fields that the resident may wish to follow and in which they can get some training. Further development of the project may be worked on after the residency is completed. Sometimes placement at specific universities or offices is conditioned on the type or format of the supported research.

1. Name of rotation: Research rotation, grant writing rotation, external funding, external financing, entrepreneurship.
2. Faculty monitor/manager: Forensic pathologist program director.
   a. Qualifications: Forensic path boards with appointment to the position of facility manager and/or resident overseer.
3. Place and facility: Residents are placed in active research labs and guided into a problem area; the rotation may be divided into work in several labs, which will extend the experience.
4. Forensic workload: The resident is introduced to the various formats of forensic research including experimental pathology, immunohistochemistry, DNA screenings, chromosomal studies, and applications of any of the forensic sciences.
5. Evidentiary product: The resident should show that they have studied the skills in research grant writing and have actively participated in the write-up of the research they are monitoring. Reports and consultations are recorded and logged.
6. Current methodology: There are no specific guidelines to be followed in selecting a research topic or area; the research should stay within the safety limitations of the laboratory.
7. Necessary skills: Creative thinking, clear written expression, solid scientific base, research team adaptability, patience and honesty.

8. Laboratory equipment: The resident should learn the principles of management of laboratory equipment with time spent on purchasing agreements, installation and maintenance of electronic and mechanical systems, equipment safety rules, engineering maintenance, and disposal problems.
9. Recording equipment: A review of the available recording equipment for each of the research disciplines is applicable to this rotation.
10. Safety discipline: A review of the safety program for the laboratory and its applied methods is needed in this rotation.

The research rotation ensures that the resident understands the continuity of membership in specialized organizations, which allows development of special skills, the use of these skills in associated research, the presentation of the research at the meetings of the organization, and the publication of the research in journals of the association.

I remember my surprise when I was called by an editor and asked to submit a pathology paper on a topic fitting a special issue of her journal. I was pleased to fulfill this need, and for me it opened a new view of scientific progress. Know thy editor.

Public Health and Environmental Health Rotation

In most jurisdictions, sudden deaths at home and work are certified by the medical examiner or the coroner. The cases of epidemic and infectious disease are also managed by the local public health organization. Although the relationships of these organizations may vary in degree and in detail, the autopsy work is the work of the forensic pathologist. The work of the public health laboratory and its officers is covered in this rotation, and the residents learn the relationship between the two offices. Environmental laws have become more federal and the management is more defined by federal agencies. In many states the attorney general has a monitoring staff that maintains active review of the functioning of nursing homes and facilities for the aged and the handicapped/impaired.

1. Name of rotation: Public health and environmental health.
2. Faculty monitor/manager: The managing scientist of the local public health laboratory, the local monitoring agents of the Department of Natural Resources, the monitoring personnel of the Attorney General's Office.
   a. Qualifications: Appointed governmental officials functioning as scientists.
3. Place and facility: Local public health laboratories.

4. Forensic workload: Cases of sudden unexpected death, environmental disaster deaths, acute and sudden infectious deaths.
5. Evidentiary product: The health lab will identify the agents of epidemic and/or sudden death. Reports and consultations are logged.
6. Current methodology: Up to date microbiological analysis of tissues and fluids; environmental studies as required.
7. Necessary skills: Laboratory management skills; diagnostic bench-work skills.
8. Laboratory equipment: A well-equipped modern laboratory with a short turnaround, a good record of accomplishment, appropriate inspections and certifications, with a monitored safe environment.
9. Recording equipment: Photography, video, and radio, with court-room presentation and enactment capability.
10. Safety discipline: The lab is able to fulfill all of the criteria for the complete growth and isolation of class 5 organisms (the deadliest); skilled and certified technical staff.

Military Forensic Pathology Rotation (Optional)

Many portions of the art and science of forensic pathology are begun and matured by the military experience before application into the civilian world. The Armed Forces Institute of Pathology (AFIP) in Washington DC was a major center for American forensic pathology. Under the leadership of several generations of great AFIP directors (Frank Townsend, MD, for example), the academic work for forensic pathology was undertaken. The AFIP loaned teaching slide sets, gave weekly and monthly courses in all aspects of pathology stressing anatomical and forensic pathology, provided consultative expertise in all areas of military and civilian pathology, developed the science of traumatic pathology, and formulated attention to the phenomenon of aircraft accidents. As the military assumed a worldwide service stance, the AFIP provided parallel development of international consultational expertise. The scientific work of the AFIP was always first class and beyond recall. The major service medical centers had active forensic pathology services and provide experience in forensic pathology historically used to qualify service veterans to provide forensic services (e.g., the autopsy of President Kennedy).

Visits to adjacent military bases may provide supportive experience in the administrative management of difficult and unusual problems.

1. Name of rotation: Military forensic pathology.
2. Faculty monitor/manager: A staff pathologist with military experience and knowledge of military medicine.
   a. Qualifications: Satisfactory completion of a military tour.

3. Place and facility: The morgue facilities of a local military base may be an effective theater for this rotational experience. Au contraire, the AFIP pathology residents would rotate at the State of Maryland Medical Examiner's Office for experience in shooting fatalities and other forensic cases.

4. Forensic workload: Since the civilian sector is also using military armament, the observational tasks of shooting homicides are no different in the civilian world than the military world. The difference is the frequency of occurrence. The military workload is more regulated and defined with different standards than the civilian.

5. Evidentiary product: The military has different legal standards than does the civilian court system; it is a military justice system. Reports and consultations are logged.

6. Current methodology: The military uses its federal laboratory system to achieve its evidentiary statements, and internal quality controls are utilized.

7. Necessary skills: The resident pathologist uses this year of monitored autopsy experience to learn the nuances and fine points of forensic anatomy dissection and histological/cytological visualization. Military cases often include mutilated and severely damaged bodies with the chance of live ammunition in the corpse. Body contamination with radiation, active chemicals, and agents of biological warfare are real possibilities in military autopsies.

8. Laboratory equipment: Includes the capacity to shield and isolate the damaged, spoiled, and contaminated (chemical molecules, physical and biological agents).

9. Recording equipment: Photography, video, and radio, with courtroom presentation and enactment capability.

10. Safety discipline: Safety discipline is a major learning responsibility in military forensic pathology.

Forensic Biology and Entomology Rotation

A review of the uses of forensic biology with forensic consultants is a valuable intellectual trip for the forensic pathology resident. The principles of time expenditure depending on the known growth rate of various insect population characteristics is explained and studied. *Essential Forensic Biology* by Alan Gunn (John Wiley & Sons, 2006) on forensic biology provides important guidelines, references, and laboratory tips for the profitable use of this discipline. It bears reading.

One of the difficulties with forensic biology and other nonforensic adjunctive sciences is the failure to follow the classic forensic topics, derivatives, or chapter headings when publishing. Forensic materials are generally classified by the type of crime and modus operandi of the criminal. Books and writings without this forensic outlook require some manipulation by the forensic reader.

1. Name of rotation: Forensic biology including forensic entomology.
2. Faculty monitor/manager: A board-certified forensic pathologist.
   a. Qualifications: Capability of using biological evidence in case solution or analysis.
3. Place and facility: A contractable biologist or forensic entomologist laboratory.
4. Forensic workload: Trace and routine case evidence analyzed with biological principles of analysis.
5. Evidentiary product: The forensic biology report as a separate or integrated report.
6. Current methodology: Applied scientific principles from biology, chemistry, physics, and the basic medical sciences presented in a referenced report.
7. Necessary skills: Biologist, experimental pathologist, surgeon.
8. Laboratory equipment: Attention is paid in Gunn's last chapter to the collection of biological materials for forensic purposes.
9. Recording equipment.
10. Safety discipline.

For most forensic pathologists, their encounters with forensic entomologists is at meetings of the American Academy of Forensic Sciences where the pathology and biology disciplines share a common section of the academy. Demonstrations of services and the associated techniques by local forensic entomology practitioners in association with any case consultations would be an appropriate learning experience for the pathology resident.

Transportation Pathology Rotation

The transportation pathology rotation is usually not separated from the routine forensic autopsy caseload. It provides a common case for most beginning residents. Some autopsy groups always start their beginners on the traffic cases. But these cases are anything but simple in analysis. In all cases where there is a substantiated diagnosis of drunk driving, the case will go to court and withstand courtroom evaluation. The autopsy diagnosis page is oftentimes the most expletive document in the death report. A review of the papers in the engineering section of the AAFS will provide valuable supplemental understanding of transportation problems.

1. Name of rotation: Transportation (motor vehicle, airplane, helicopter, boats and water transportation), bicycle, pediatric transportation (e.g., baby buggy, car seat), geriatric transportation (e.g., wheelchair, body lifts), trucks, and transporters.
2. Faculty monitor/manager: An experienced forensic pathologist with mechanical engineering interests/education.
   a. Qualifications: Board certification and engineering experience; concurrent community safety training.
3. Place and facility: Industrial and road accident scene experience.
4. Forensic workload: Roadway deaths on regulated and nonregulated roads (e.g., farming, hunting, and mining), which are usually worked by the state police rather than local police forces. Car bombings may be studied here or in the homicide section.
5. Evidentiary product: An incident report, photographs, autopsy report, toxicology, trace evidence (e.g., clothing, air-bag evidence), consultations.
6. Current methodology: Cell phone photography, dictated scene reports, blood alcohol testing, Mothers Against Drunk Driving (MADD) protocols, scene interviews.
7. Necessary skills: Knowledge of local alcoholism and drug standards and community expectations, vehicular evidence (air bag, frame distortions, light and instrument panel crash changes).
8. Laboratory equipment: Complete forensic lab with microscopy and computer support.
9. Recording equipment: Photography, video, and radio, with courtroom presentation and enactment capability.
10. Safety discipline: A fire department presence is required in most transportation accidents to control the fuel problems; registration of dangerous/explosive/volatile loads is required. A wide scene parameter may be required and neighborhoods evacuated.

Forensic Pathology Office Management Rotation (Visiting Other Training Sites and Forensic Offices)

The forensic pathology office management rotation is a self-directed tour of the local and regional forensics offices, which may have employment opportunities and provide an alternative viewpoint of forensic pathology not presented in the one-year program the resident has experienced. In one week's time at least five offices can be visited and compared. The selection of offices (tour schedule) allows the residency director to send students to the available local savants of the profession at the time of residency completion. The tour may be varied in its scheduling and interrelated with meeting appointments.

Forensic Odontology Rotation (May Be Required When Odontology Is Not Included in the Autopsy Rotation)

1. Name of rotation: Forensic odontology.
2. Faculty monitor/manager: A dentist or forensic pathologist with forensic dentistry teaching capability.
   a. Qualifications: Forensic experience in identification and bite case analysis.
3. Place and facility: Residency training facility and morgue.
4. Forensic workload: Living and deceased dental description and formal forensic identification analysis of human dental arcades at all ages and in all forensic circumstances. Consultations with police authorities, lawyers, and prosecutors.
5. Evidentiary product: Written description and analytical forensic dentistry report with supportive DNA, photographic, scan, and radiology evidence.
6. Current methodology: Each autopsy will use a case-specific dental identification system. The extent of description will match the extent of the dental data on the study and closing of the case. A summative sentence description may be used, whereas in cases in which identification is a major concern, the dental description can be descriptive anatomically (each tooth is numbered and described) with adjunctive photography and radiology. Animal bite characteristics and DNA analytical techniques are practiced.
7. Necessary skills: Basic knowledge of dental description methods, the anatomy of the teeth and the age changes of the dental arcades, and the forensic utility of forensic prosthetic devices. Knowledge of current identification technology including fingerprinting, iridal pattern recognition, radiological, and bite-mark technology and analysis, including patterned injury analysis.
8. Laboratory equipment: Crowbars and spreading jaw openers, mirrors, dental hand tools (probes, scissors, pliers, wires, dissecting equipment, wires, hammers, chisels), scanning and radiography equipment, imprint and casting supplies, DNA and genetic sampling kits.
9. Recording equipment: Photography and radiology (still and scan) equipment.
10. Safety discipline: Conventional and infectious disease precautions and behavior with active safety monitoring.

Clinical Forensic Pathology Rotation

The clinical forensic pathology rotation includes pathologist service in many different settings in the entire cooperative community including prisons and jails, street crime scenes, emergency rooms, intensive care and immediate care facilities in hospitals and emergency medical facilities where acute and delayed trauma lesion identification and evaluation is recorded scientifically and given appropriate timing, comatose patient triage and management techniques, patient identification and interviewing with controlled language facilities, psychiatric patient support with drug evaluation, immigrant problems with toxicology and infectious disease monitoring, domestic dispute injury and clinical pathology evaluation, service to the community hospice program in the service area with defined identification and staging of the fatal disease states considered operative in the hospice patients, the many aspects of gun availability and gun control in the service area, parenting problems, childhood injury evaluations and summations, police prisoner management including illegal drug availability, restraint training and standards, and taser gun deaths as initial areas facilitating appropriate training. The resident is taught the appropriate protocol in the patient problem areas related to forensic pathology and his or her ability to identify causative factors and active pathological processes.

Clinical forensic pathology is an underrepresented clinical service area in this country. As a consequence, much of the identifiable and useable evidence is not presented in legal or medical case presentation. Most important is the loss of accurate description of the forensic signs and symptoms arising in the initial period of active hospitalization and emergency treatment. Active participation of many attending specialists will be required to present an adequate program.

Active programs are present in Orlando, Florida, with William Anderson, MD.

Bibliography

Gunn, A. *Essential Forensic Biology*. Chichester, UK: Wiley, 2006.

Zohn, H. K., Dashow, S., Aschheim, K. W., Dobrin, L. A., Glazer, H. K., Kirschbaum, M., Levitt, D., and Feldman, C. A. The odontology victim identification skill assessment system. *Journal of Forensic Science* 55, no. 3 (2010): 788–791.

Forensic Pathology Essentials   III

In this part, the essentials are presented with a code. Learning objectives as essentials are distinguished by an M or an S

- The M after an objective relates it as a memorized fact or concept. ("This you must know." —John Egletis, MD, Ohio State University professor)
- The S after an objective relates to a manual or physical skill. This you must do. Please self-assess your motor skills carefully.

Just as musicians have a play list, forensic pathologists have a fact list and a skill list. These are the essences of our profession. Know your objectives.

The Governmental Role in Forensic Pathology

3

Training in forensic pathology is generally fashioned through the government and its agencies; training in the forensic work carried out in the private sector is unscheduled. The training relates to and its availability is dependent upon the outside activities of the teaching staff at the residency institution.

Private consulting work is considered advanced in complexity and so it is not considered topically proper for initial training in forensic pathology. Some programs immediately place their residents into private casework. Private casework is any autopsy performed outside the usual jurisdiction of the teaching office.

Who actually runs the government office? Regardless of the legislative intent in formulating a political body to handle the problem of public death, the systems vary from site to site and from system to system, that is, whether the format is as a medical examiner system with a forensic pathologist in charge or a coroner's system with a forensic pathologist as a consultant doctor. The circumstances of leadership and who gives the orders may not be well defined. The forensic pathologist may find himself or herself taking directions in some matters from the scene investigator, the chief secretary, the office manager, the police at the scene or at the autopsy, the lab manager, the chief investigator, the department chair in universities, the elected coroner, the appointed chief medical examiner or his or her delegate, someone from the district attorney's office, a board chairman or member, or another police agency (FBI, or state agency associates). It depends on the leadership style and method of the person in charge of the agency.

I once had the pleasure of running a College of American Pathologists (CAP) lab inspection and I discovered that the woman in charge of the lab had the minimal lab training of a laboratory aide. But she was laboratory wise and a clever person with things and people, so after eight or ten years of working in the lab she was the best at administration and lab analysis in the group of twenty-five to thirty people. Over the years she had acquired the necessary certification and training for the lab leadership position and she did it well. So much for the PhD and doctorate degree in the medical lab. Home cooking works.

Political correctness and ethical considerations are important when dealing with government agencies and related organizations.

Objectives

1. Delineate the relationship and the progression of the Napoleonic code to the development of modern death investigation. M
2. Give several examples of proper (legal) involvement of the government in the investigation of death and give several examples of abusive situations in the investigation of death. M
3. Describe the role that some medical examiners play in the circumstance of cerebral comatose death. M
4. Compare the English common law coroner's system to the Napoleonic medical examiner's system of central Europe. M
5. Identify the following persons from the preceding forensic generation:

Vernard Adams, MD	R. B. H. Gradwohl, MD
Lester Adelson, MD	Michael Graham, MD
Michael M. Baden, MD	Ali Hameli, MD
Andrew M. Baker, MD	Randy Hanzlick, MD
Millard Bass, DO	Christopher Happy, MD
Phillip Burch, MD	Richard Harruff, MD
John D. Butts, MD	Milton Helpern, MD
F. E. Camp, MD	Gordon Hennigar, MD
Joye Carter, MD	Charles Hirsch, MD
Mary Case, MD	Donald R. Jason, MD
J. Caspir, MD	Nancy L. Jones, MD
Richard Childs, LLB	Deborah Kay, MD
John Coe, MD	Ron Kornblum, MD
Tracey Corey, MD	E. Kowolski, MD
Greg Davis, MD	Emil Laga, MD
Joseph Davis, MD	Patrick E. Lantz, MD
Lance G. Davis, MD	Charles Larson, MD
Stanley Durlacher, MD	Timothy Leary, PhD
Bill Eckert, MD	Frances Glessner Lee
J. Felo, DO	James L. Luke, MD
Russell Fisher, MD	Geoffrey Mann, MD
Richard Ford, MD	K. Mant, MD
David R. Fowler, MD	Ann Martin, MD
Richard C. Froede, MD	George McGrath
James L. Frost, MD	F. P. Miller III, MD
Randall Frost, MD	A. R. Moritz, MD
George Gantner, MD	Thomas Naguchi, MD
Jan Garavaglia, MD	Jefferey Nine, MD
Samuel Gerber, MD	Charles Norris, MD
J. Glaister, MD	Joshua A. Perper, MD

Edith Potter, MD
Clara Raven, MD
C. Schandl, MD
Barry Scheck, LLB
Carl Schmidt, MD
Oscar Schultz, MD
A. Shakir, MD
Ronald Singer, MS
Daniel Spitz, MD
Werner Spitz, MD
William Sturner, MD

M. Trotter, PhD
Jane Turner, MD
S. Turner, MD
T. Tworek, MD
M. Vance, MD
E. Von Hamm, MD
Cyril H. Wecht, MD
Dwayne A. Wolf, MD
James Young, MD
Ross Zumwalt, MD

6. Define the role of the probate judge in the scheme of death investigation. Compare death with a will, death with a trust, and death with no will. M
7. Explain the relationship of the medical examiner/coroner to the undertaker and undertaker societies/organizations. M
8. Define the jurisdiction of a case and describe several instances where the jurisdiction becomes a factor in the death investigation. M
9. What is the role of the coroner/medical examiner in the property of the deceased? Discuss the property issue involving aliens and travelers. M
10. From what source does the coroner/medical examiner derive authority for his actions? M
11. Under what circumstances does a hospital autopsy become a medicolegal autopsy? M
12. Define the relationship of the medical examiner/coroner to the authority and jurisdiction of the following government agencies. Also what is the role of the coroner/medical examiner Web site in these relationships? M

> Army, Marines, Navy, Air Force, and Coast Guard
> Immigration service
> Local police, sheriff, social workers, attorney general
> Occupational Safety and Health Administration (OSHA)
> State highway patrol
> Department of Justice, Federal Bureau of Investigation (FBI)
> Centers for Disease Control and Prevention's Medical Examiner/
> Coroner Information Sharing Program (MecISP)
> Civil Aeronautics Board, local airfield safety
> Department of Energy
> Fire departments
> Local and state medical boards

State pharmaceutical board, federal Drug Enforcement Administration (DEA)

Governor and elected officials

What is the role of the coroner/ME website in these relationships?

13. Review the information required for the complete fulfillment of a death certificate. What items present formidable problems with the available software programs in use today? M

14. Relate the completion of the death certificate and its problems to the functioning and jurisdiction of the coroner/medical examiner. M

15. Define the relationship of the department of health (or equivalent) to the medical examiner/coroner. Explain the use of the public health laboratory in fulfilling the microbiological needs of the medical examiner/coroner. Relate the economic demands of epidemics on both organizations. M

16. Discuss the relationship of military service deaths in a civilian milieu to their civilian certification and how the military functions in these cases. M

17. What problems arise at the international borders? How are boundaries defined in the maritime service? M

18. Define the problem of death as related to the following problems: M
Dried bones found in a desert
Bodies found in tar pits or bogs
Decomposed bodies lacking any identification data

19. Discuss the relationship of the medical examiner/coroner with fetal death certification. M

20. Discuss the role of the medical examiner/coroner in the definition of death in missing persons cases. M

21. Discuss the role of the coroner/medical examiner in the deaths caused by the abuse of the legitimate pharmacological industry. Discuss the role of the licensing agencies. Indicate the extent of this problem in the United States. M

22. What are the legal supports of the coroner/medical examiner in his/her jurisdiction? How is the coroner/medical examiner protected and what are his/her areas of vulnerability? M

23. Demonstrate the completion of a death certificate in the following circumstances of death: S
Accidental death
Natural death
Suicide
Pending completion
Homicide

24. Discuss the role of the computer in the medical examiner's/coroner's office in regard to: M

> Maintenance of records and federal government standards
> Searches
> Police communication

25. Discuss the role of the medical examiner/coroner system in the development of trace element technology. M
26. Describe the death investigation scheme used in the study of environmental contamination, using mercury as an example. M
27. Describe the characteristics of each of the major periods of American forensic pathology:

> 1840–1929, the detective period (the English model with the dominant role of the insane asylum and capital punishment)
> 1929–1963, the scientific period (immigrant physicians and toxicologists from Hitler's Europe)
> 1963–1990, the medical expert period (the American Academy of Forensic Sciences directory)
> 1990–2009, the heroic television period (Note: Elizabeth Devine, a former crime scene investigator and a niece of Dr. Ronald Kornblum, a former chief medical examiner for Los Angeles County, California, carries the details of forensic pathology into the homes of America as a writer with the *CSI: Crime Scene Investigation* series.)

28. Detail the presidential assassination autopsies of Kennedy, Lincoln, and Garfield. Discuss the death circumstances and autopsy of Bobby Kennedy following a hotel shooting in Los Angeles, California.

Vocabulary

Accidental death
Death in custody
Death on the job
Elder abuse
Environmental hazards
Homicide by drugs
Illegal abortion
Maintenance of records
Medical malpractice
Misplaced evidence
Natural death
Pending completion
Police communication
Police communication guidelines
Searches

Searches in police custody
Sexual assault
Suicide
Survivors of suicide
Trace element technology
Vehicular trauma

Bibliography

Books and Articles

Corrigan, G. E. Public death: A basic philosophical concept of forensic pathology and medicine. *Journal of Forensic Sciences* 20, no. 1 (1975): 154–158.

Kubler-Ross, E. *On Death and Dying: What the Living Have to Teach Doctors, Nurses, Clergy and Their Own Families.* New York: MacMillan, 1969.

Ferguson, W. R. *Technician's Guide for Postmortem Examinations.* Bloomington, IN: Xlibris, 2010.

Hanzlick, R., ed. *Cause of Death and Death Certification: Important Information for Physicians, Medical Examiners, Coroners, and the Public.* Northfield, IL: College of American Pathologists, 2006.

Periodicals

Evidence Technology Magazine. www.evidencemagazine.com. Dedicated to the technology of evidence collection, processing, and preservation.

Forensic Science: Policy & Management. An international quarterly journal that discusses current laboratory and scientist issues.

Organizations

American Academy of Forensic Sciences, www.aafs.org
American Board of Criminalistics, www.criminalistics.com
American Board of Forensic Anthropology, www.theabfa.org
American Board of Forensic Document Examiners, www.abfde.org
American Board of Forensic Toxicology, www.abft.org
American Board of Pathology, www.abpath.org
American Board of Psychiatry and Neurology, www.abpn.com
American Society of Clinical Pathologists, www.ascp.org
College of American Pathologists, www.cap.org
International Board of Forensic Engineering Science, www.iifes.org
National Association of Medical Examiners, www.thename.org
National Expert Witness Conference, www.SEAK.com
Pathology Outlines, www.pathologyoutlines.org
World Health Organization *World Report on Violence and Health*, www.who.int

The Medical Examiner and Coroner Systems with Comparisons and Evaluations

4

(Note: The variance of comparative systems for public death management has never been an issue in the recent federal elections.)

Objectives

1. Compare the medical examiner and coroner systems; discuss the difference between being an elected official and an appointed official. M
2. Discuss the methods of appointment in common use today. Describe testing methods. M
3. Compare the differences between a pathologist working in a state-authorized system, a county system, a city system, and a military system. Compare and contrast statewide coroner systems with statewide medical examiner systems. M
4. Discuss the development and use of the coroner's court. M
5. Discuss the mechanisms that replace the coroner's court in the medical examiner system model. M
6. Discuss the impounding of a coroner's jury and the conditions under which hearings are held in the coroner's system. M
7. Discuss the powers of subpoena of the medical examiner and the coroner in the two systems and how the power is used. M
8. Discuss the relationship of the judiciary to the coroner system, and compare and contrast this with the relationship of the judiciary to the medical examiner. M
9. Discuss the social and political forces that limit the utilization of the autopsy. M
10. Discuss the international situation in relationship to the procurement and utilization of the autopsy. Consider the Middle East and the Muslim world. M
11. Discuss the malpractice problems of the medical examiner. M
12. Contrast the medical examiner malpractice problems with those of a coroner. M
13. Discuss the testimonial character of physicians working in the medical examiner's office as contrasted with those working in the coroner's jurisdiction. M

14. Compare and contrast the most successful coroner's systems with the most successful medical examiner's systems prevalent today. M
15. Compare and contrast the judiciary powers of the coroner with those of the medical examiner. M
16. Discuss the limitations of the nonmedically trained coroner in contrast to the medically trained coroner. M
17. Discuss the role of the trained physician's assistant and pathologist assistant in a modern medical examiner's system. M
18. Discuss the role of the lay investigator in modern forensic investigation. M
19. What are the limits and the prerogatives of laymen in death investigation? M
20. Compare and contrast local environmental and sociological idioms in the investigation of death. M
21. Enumerate the property handling functions within a modern medical examiner's office. M
22. Describe the International Association of Coroners & Medical Examiners. M
23. Discuss the role of the coroner's referee. M
24. Draw a table of organization of a medical examiner's office. M
25. Draw a table of organization (personnel) of a coroner's office. M
26. Indicate a standard type of budget for a coroner's office and for a medical examiner's office. M
27. Describe the required body handling capabilities of a medical examiner's or coroner's office. M
28. What are the associated problems in body storage? Cremains storage? M
29. Discuss the administrative personnel problems related to the civil service regulations at the city, county, and state levels. M
30. Discuss the record handling problems encountered in a medical examiner's and a coroner's office. What are the leading software programs filling this activity? M
31. Detail the paper flow of a case from the time of discovery of the body to the closing of the case with burial or cremation. M
32. Discuss the role of the statistician in the medical examiner's office and detail the items necessary for a yearly report. M
33. Delineate the problems with the official recognition and identification of corpses and indicate the methods for solving them. M
34. Discuss the role of the diener staff in the management of the medical examiner's or coroner's office. M
35. Draw a floor plan for a medical examiner's office morgue to include airflow, lighting, analytical instrumentation, cadaver storage facilities, dissection areas, forensic science space, personal hygiene

facilities, storage space, communications facilities, and office space. M

36. Draw an expandable floor plan for a county medical examiner's office and morgue facility. Include communications equipment and facilities. M

37. Indicate the necessary adjuncts of a state system beyond the maintenance of a county system of service. M

38. Relate the role of the state medical examiner to other elected and appointed officials. M

39. Delineate the methods of appointment and control of a state medical examiner. M

40. Discuss the methods of funding of medical examiner/coroner systems. M

41. Discuss the relationship of the state health laboratory to the state medical examiner office and its laboratories. M

42. Discuss the role of the medical examiner system in the investigation of sex crimes. M

43. Relate the medical examiner's office to the social welfare system. M

44. Discuss the methods of making case decisions in a medical examiner's office; relate the overviewing role of the chief medical examiner to the work of the other medical examiners. M

45. Discuss the evidentiary techniques of the medical examiner's office in developing a case and relate these techniques to the areas of property maintenance, personal identification, and the development of trace evidence with and without microscopy. M

46. Discuss the role of public relations in the functioning of the medical examiner's office. Relate the use of the Internet and collaboration with television stations in the solution of medical examiner problems. M

47. Compare and contrast the judiciary/legal capabilities of a coroner with medical scientific capacities of a medical examiner. Indicate the role of the increasing size of the caseload in limiting the extent and depth of case evaluation. M

48. Discuss the sociopolitical problem of *nativism*. Relate the differences in public management in the various regions of the United States. Relate the differences between elected and appointed public officials. M

49. Discuss the problems and expenses of cremation. Relate the death certificate problems of cremation. M

50. Describe and discuss the courtroom appearances of the coroner and/or the medical examiner. M

51. Discuss the role of the pathologist as a consultant to either the state or the defense at the primary trial level, or appellate level. M

52. Discuss the methods available to respond to legal questions. M

53. Identify the various roles of the dentist in the activities of the medical examiner's office. What equipment and facilities are needed? M
54. Discuss the utilization of the "outside" reference laboratory in the provision of a fully described and studied scientific case study. M
55. Discuss the role of federal laboratories in the maintenance of complete case coverage. M
56. Discuss the relationship of a medical examiner's/coroner's office to the university complex. M
57. Discuss the problems arising in the university affiliation and the academic recognition of the forensic pathologist/coroner. M
58. Discuss the methods for developing new disciplinary interactions in a medical examiner/coroner system. M
59. Discuss the role of the double signing of autopsy protocols and utilization of absentee witnesses in court testimonials. M
60. Discuss the utilization of the grand jury in forensic cases. M
61. Discuss the development of the medical examiner system in the United States after World War II. Describe the 1954 Model Post-Mortem Examinations Act and its effects in Oregon and the city of Chicago. M
62. Describe the evolution of the forensic morgue and the associated elements of the forensic sciences from the community medical laboratory to the large regional forensic center capable of the autopsy, forensic pathology, toxicology, anthropology, trace evidence, and radiology. How did the forensic morgue arise from the hospital laboratory in terms of leadership, academic personnel, elected officials, additional scientists, and forensic scientists? How did anthropology and toxicology merge with forensic pathology? Was there a common political pattern of connection or was the pattern dictated by local conditions?

Vocabulary

Assembly and delegates
Body disposal
Business approaches to the practice of science
Complete autopsy
Inspection and examination
Investment return
Mass fatalities
Protocol and key performance indicators
Regulations and standards
Tissue donation

Bibliography

Book

DiMaio, V. J., and DiMaio, D. *Forensic Pathology*. 2nd ed. Boca Raton, FL: CRC Press, 2001.

Periodical

Forensic Science: Policy & Management. A new journal, published by Taylor & Francis, on the business and policy of forensic science to include best practices, policy with recommendations, science education and training, economics, quality control, staffing, process improvements, budgeting, ethics, and legal relationships.

Organization

Advance for Administrators of the Laboratory, www.advanceweb.com, www.anylabtestnow.com. An inexpensive franchise system for ambulatory to storefront sales of medical and forensic laboratory testing.

Research, Development, and Evaluation Programs

Criminal justice statistical programs have collections of various studies with the associated numerical data. Also the Forensic Resource Network was created by the National Institute of Justice to help local and state forensic laboratories with training; technology transfer; methods of research, development, testing, and evaluation; and analytical services. Network members include Marshall University forensics, University of Central Florida, National Forensic Science Technology Center, and West Virginia University forensics.

The Academic
Discipline of
Forensic Pathology

5

Forensic pathology has been poorly represented in U.S. medical education ever since Harvard University and its School of Medicine dropped its distinguished School of Legal Medicine in 1966. Charles S. Petty, MD, a Harvard graduate and a great teacher at the University of Maryland and later chief medical examiner for Dallas County, Texas, was ready for the position but was denied the chair as the School of Legal Medicine closed.

As a consequence, the Massachusetts Medical Examiner Office was weakened and underwent periodic times of turmoil. No other school took Harvard's premier place in educational leadership. But most schools followed Harvard's example and went from a service format with populist care for the designated population in their precinct to active pursuit of research dollars. Teachers now were judged by the amount of their grants and not the number or quality of their students.

The Armed Forces Institute of Pathology (AFIP) took a major role in forensic education and the New York, Philadelphia, Baltimore, Los Angeles, and Miami offices were leaders in the post-WWII era. The loss of the Harvard school was a deadly blow to academic forensic pathology. Several of the new and old state medical examiner systems, including New Mexico and Florida, provided leadership, but the academic progress of the post-WWII era was related more to the presence of strong intelligent forensic pathologists who were good scientists and writers than to a strong economically based home office conjoined with an academic department. Economic support was a problem (the patients are dead and no one will charge the estate of the dead person, although the business began as a method of raising taxes for the king!) and funding for forensic research was nonexistent. As a result, compared to other scientists, U.S. forensic scientists have had limited achievements in the past half century. One recent census of U.S. forensic path students (residents) enrollment was placed only at twenty-five for the year 2010.

The National Institutes of Health (NIH) was not a player in forensic science economics. The American Board of Pathology followed a role of passive certifier of expertise and provided an examination venue for a diverse set of training programs. It gave honest, reliable, standardized, and applicable examinations. The Federal Bureau of Investigation (FBI) was without academic connection and had little forensic scientific competition. However, the FBI led the country into many new areas of forensic science. Recently, a council of educators has been formed by the American Academy of Forensic Sciences (AAFS) and is initiating needed reforms. The American Board of Pathology has been maintained as the major administrative tool of forensic pathology specialty recognition by its certification procedures.

In essence, the massive progressive influx of governmental funds into medical research was not funneled into forensic research but into the monetary stakes of drug research, aided and abetted by the medical school research establishment.

Objectives

1. Discuss the origin of the subspecialty of forensic pathology and its certification with the American Board of Pathology. What is the role of the American Medical Association? M
2. Outline the format for the subspecialty examination in forensic pathology. M
3. Delineate the procedures necessary to become an examiner member on the forensic board. M
4. Discuss the development of other specialties in the forensic sciences, including the boards in toxicology and physical anthropology. M
5. Delineate the role of the federal government and the Law Enforcement Alliance of America (LEAA) in the formation of subspecialty boards. M
6. Discuss the advantages of a board system and relate its disadvantages to the advantages. M
7. Describe the typical one-year or two-year program in forensic pathology training. Outline its major objectives. M
8. Enumerate the most important training areas and offices in forensic pathology. Give a brief contemporary history of each office. M
9. Discuss the role of the forensic pathologist as an administrator of a medical legal office. What is the role of the nonmedical administrator in a medical examiner's office? M
10. Give a breakdown of the major medical and scientific associations in forensic pathology. M
11. Note those associations that sponsor original research at their meetings. M
12. Name several areas of progress in forensic pathology since WWII. M
13. Discuss the relationship of training in hospital pathology to the daily activities of the forensic pathologist. M
14. Enumerate the leading texts in the discipline of forensic pathology. What are the leading Internet sites? M

15. Enumerate the leading journals in the discipline of forensic pathology. What are the leading forensic journal Web sites? M

16. Discuss the use of the community radiological diagnostic services in the analysis of forensic patients. Comment on the evolution of the CAT scan into forensics. M

17. Discuss the use of histology and special staining methods in forensic pathology. What methods of quality control are available? How should these services be budgeted? M

18. Discuss the limitations in the determination of the time of death. How is the taking of the temperature of the dead body properly managed and recorded? M

19. What are the limitations (limiting factors) of central nervous system analysis in forensic pathology? Discuss the attributes and problems of immediate brain dissection at the time of autopsy. M

20. Discuss the coding methods currently available in forensic pathology and delineate its terminology. Are autopsies part of the Medicare program? M

21. Identify the following and explain the current use in forensic practice: M

    International Classification of Diseases (ICD)
    Systematized Nomenclature of Medicine (SNOMED)
    Systematized Nomenclature of Medicine—Clinical Terms
        (SNOMED CT)
    Current procedural terminology
    Systematized Nomenclature of Pathology (SNOP)
    International classification of disease (WHO International)

22. Discus the heritage of forensic pathology with its British Isles derivation and derivatives from continental sources such as France, Germany, and Vienna. How did the forensic services evolve in the Muslim and Hindu worlds? M

23. Discuss the interface of forensic pathology with the following societal activities: M

    Law and the police
    University and the medical school
    Law school and the judiciary
    Government and the attorney general's office
    Church and the cemetery

24. Enumerate the major research technologies available within the laboratory disciplines of forensic pathology. M

25. Indicate the types of research directly under the direction of the forensic pathologist and those that are directed in accompaniment with other scientists. M

26. Identify recognized forensic scientists in criminology, pathology, and other forensic areas from the following countries and regions: M

> United States
> Canada
> Mexico
> Latin America
> Caribbean
> British Isles
> Continental Europe
> Russia
> Middle East
> India
> China
> Japan
> Singapore
> Southeast Asia
> Australia

27. Discuss the role of the state police and the police surgeon in the South American development of forensic pathology. M

28. Identify some of the leading sites on the Internet for the forensic sciences and forensic literature. Describe the available literary services (management of text downloading) and their cost. M

29. Enumerate the various academic degrees in forensic science and forensic pathology. M

30. Discuss the value, utility, resourcefulness, cost, availability and effectiveness of graduate education on the Web. State some examples of Web educational efforts. M

Vocabulary

Certification and registration
County coroner
Evaluation and identification
Fraud
Misdemeanor
State associations of coroners
State attorney general oversight duties
State medical examiner systems
Web education

Bibliography

Standard forensic pathology texts in print can be found using www. Amazon.com and other online search engines. Vincent J. DiMaio and Dominick DiMaio, Werner Spitz, and David Dolinak are popular authors. A visit to the AAFS annual meeting is effective in keeping up with the industry. A great general science meeting is Pittcon (www.pittcon.org), the largest conference and exposition for laboratory science. Newcomers to forensic pathology and the forensic sciences need to review the AAFS annual set of abstracts of the papers presented at its meeting, the Proceedings of the American Academy of Forensic Sciences. It is an inch thick and has up-to-date addresses for the forensic scientists with abstracts of their current work.

Also, I use Google and Yahoo search engines to send me daily e-mail on the subjects of medical examiner, forensic autopsy, forensic pathology, and coroner. I monitor at least 30 forensic news stories a day. If it happens, I know about it.

Books

Dolinak, D., Matshes, E., and Lew, E. *Forensic Pathology: Principles and Practice*. San Diego, CA: Elsevier, 2005. (Required reading for forensic pathologists to understand the systems where they will be working.)

Inman, K., and Rudin, N. *Principles and Practice of Criminalistics: The Profession of Forensic Science*. Boca Raton FL: CRC Press, 2001.

Pyrek, Kelly M. *Forensic Science Under Siege*. New York: Academic Press, 2007. (A comprehensive critical review.)

Periodicals

Evidence Technology Magazine. www.evidencemagazine.com. Technical publication for crime scene investigation units of law enforcement agencies.

Forensic Magazine. www.forensicmag.com. Technology, trends, products, and solutions for forensic professionals.

Organizations

American Academy of Forensic Sciences (AAFS), www.aafs.org. Has an annual meeting, and awards, grants, scholarships, foundations. It publishes the *Journal of Forensic Science, Academy News, Young Forensic Scientists Newsletter*. Offers ten sections: general, jurisprudence, odontology, pathology/biology, physical anthropology, psychiatry and behavioral science, questioned documents, toxicology, digital and multimedia sciences, and engineering sciences.

In addition to state pathology organizations, the following Web sites are helpful with forensic pathology information and job searches:

American Society of Clinical Pathology, www.ascp.org
College of American Pathology, www.cap.org
Indian Health Service, www.ihs.gov
National Association of Medical Examiners, www.thename.org
Pathologyoutlines.org, www.pathologyoutlines.org
U.S. Department of Veterans Affairs, www.va.gov

Scene Investigation

6

Naguchi, Baden, Zugibe, and other forensic pathologists relate their scene experiences in their personal memoirs. These are easily found and should be studied. Scene training in residency is easy as you can just ride along with the body pickup crew. Get this firsthand experience and be sure to do some of the early morning case pickups. Partnering with the police in their scene work is in all forensic programs. The current dilemma in scenes is the unrecorded (by photography) death scene that is turned into a life rescue event by emergency medical crews, often fire department groups. There is often a complete disdain for the forensic aspects of cases when confronted with a fresh collapse. Of course, that is because the firemen are directed to the lifesaving conditions of their employment. There is no forensic science supervision save for occasional irate prosecutors or homicide detectives who miss critical evidence necessary to close their cases. The coroner's office or the pathologist is given a third illegible carbon copy of the EMT report.

Scene destruction does not occur when the body is discovered by the police and considered a possible homicide. Other scenes may be more easily compromised. This is a local issue and demands continued vigilance and incident reporting.

Objectives

1. Name the major forensic texts dealing with the crime scene. Identify organizations, teaching programs, and Web sites devoted to the forensic scene. M
2. Identify the paper flow (initial and continuing reports of various portions/elements of the scene) of a proper and complete scene investigation. Include photography, spectroscopy, fingerprints, trace evidence, DNA collection, witness reports, and statements. M
3. Describe a modern system for establishing a proper scene investigation in the following localities: M
    Rural automobile accidents
    Off-road vehicular accidents
    Light aircraft accident
    Interstate vehicular accidents
    Rural homicides

Suicide with homicide, double homicides

Urban black-on-black homicide

Urban natural deaths

4. Delineate the advantages of a sound movie camera in the archival storage of a scene. M
5. Demonstrate one scene coverage by a sound camera. S
6. What are the deficiencies in the sound camera recording systems? Describe other systems of scene recording. M
7. Discuss the methods of hand drawing of the scene. M
8. Review the trace methodology available in the forensic examination of the scene. M
9. Delineate the dualistic approach of divided authority (medical examiner and police) at the scene investigation. Describe its advantages and problems. M
10. What is a police-dominated scene in comparison to a medical-examiner-dominated scene? M
11. Discuss the handling and documentation of personal property and valuables at open public scenes and closed private scenes. M
12. Delineate the activities of the medical examiner/coroner in the hospital scene and the expressed rights, duties, and obligations of the medical personnel in attendance. M
13. Discuss the axiom "the autopsy verifies the scene." M
14. Discuss the necessity of the forensic pathologist at the scene and compare it with the systems where the forensic pathologist does not go to the scene. M
15. Relate the utility of a member of the prosecutor's office assisting at the scene investigation. M
16. Discuss the limiting factors in manpower attendance and skills at the scene investigation. M
17. Describe the historic development of the lay medical examiner in the United States. M
18. Relate the major problems arising from a hasty, incomplete scene investigation. M
19. Discuss the role of the medical examiner in the distinction/recognition of "immediate suspects" in homicide cases. M
20. Identify the contents of a properly organized and equipped scene instrument and equipment container. M
21. What instruments and tools are useful in the investigation of the following special scenes? M

Automobile accidents

Motorcycle accidents

Industrial accidents

Electrocutions

Chemical poisonings
Jail deaths
Suspected homicidal poisonings

22. Discuss the role of the medical examiner in the scene investigation in cases of putrefying odoriferous bodies. What services are provided? M

23. Relate the medical examiner's activities to the maintenance of proper hygiene in putrefaction cases. M

24. Discuss the management and utilization with correlation of the evidence taken at the scene to include evidence from the medical examiner, police, fire department, social workers, and other assigned investigators including the district attorney. M

25. Discuss the subpoena powers of the medical examiner in terms of activities at a scene. Is the operating room of the hospital in which a homicide victim dies considered a part of a murder scene? Discuss the obtaining of evidence from the operation area. M

26. Discuss the role of the medical examiner in instances where the scene is destroyed, intentionally or unintentionally. M

27. Relate the manner in which proper scene management discipline may be maintained and supervised. M

28. Give an illustration of medical examiner harassment at a scene. What are the guidelines for participant photography at a scene? M

29. Discuss the relationship of the scene and its findings to the need for instantaneous press coverage of the events. M

30. Discuss the duties of the medical examiner/coroner in the instance of a scene associated with possible highly communicable and contagious diseases. M

31. Discuss the activities of the medical examiner/coroner in the instance of death at sea. M

32. Discuss the powers, responsibilities, and activities of the medical examiner/coroner in the instance of death en route in an airplane, train, or boat. M

33. Discuss the problems arising in motor transit deaths with certification occurring outside the jurisdiction of the medical examiner/coroner. M

34. Describe the appropriate specimens to be taken at the scene in contrast to those to be taken at the morgue. What is the advantage of scene-secured specimens? What is the advantage of specimens obtained at the morgue? M

35. Describe the advantages of the use of forensic entomology in scene investigation. M

36. Relate the role of the forensic botanist and the forensic anthropologist to appropriate scene investigation activities. M

37. Relate the use of soil type technology to the evidentiary search of the scene and its contents. Discuss the procurement of expert opinions on the nature of soils and soil types. M

38. Describe the usual conditions in which Native American bones are recovered. Trace a logical order of assessments that would be made over a set of these bones. M

39. Describe the procedure for procuring forensic science support for the mass examination of bodies in disaster areas. M

40. Describe the utilization of emergency refrigeration facilities for small, intermediate, and large groups of bodies. M

41. Discuss the relationship of the scene investigation to the functions and duties of the funeral director/undertaker. M

42. Discuss the relationship of the scene examiner to the variable religious factors found in the typical American population. M

43. In an industrial scene workup, how are appropriate environmental controls and samples to be taken? M

44. Describe a typical death scene related to the following crimes: M
    Sodomy with asphyxiation
    Alcoholism with falls on furniture
    Rape of a geriatric female
    Manic psychosis in a closed cell
    Epileptic furor in a domestic scene

45. Describe the scene investigation report of a fantasized (hidden and sequestered) crime. M

46. Discuss the methods of body part study and identification, and relate their entry into an appropriate forensic informatics software program. M

47. Discuss methods of scene investigation and management with very specialized forensic scene investigators; include methods and systems of marking evidence at crime scenes. M

48. Multiple crime scenes may be worked by one or many departments. Discuss the logistics of multiple scenes and how the evidence is logged and booked. M

49. Provide a protocol for management of images from security cameras located at:
    Homes
    Apartments
    Businesses
    Vehicles (cars and trucks)
    School buses and train cars
    Stores and parking lots
    Jails and police stations

50. In a multiple-scene case, how is the master list of evidence managed and protected? M
51. What are the new standards and technologies in the evidentiary use of blood alcohol measurements? M
52. Describe the differences and uses of elution and extraction in rape examination. M
53. Describe the recent technical changes in the presentation of the crime scene to a judge or jury. Discuss photography, videography, mock-up presentations, and cartoon technology. M
54. Discuss the management and numbering of crime scenes complicated with multiple investigators, multiple scenes, and multiple incidents. Identify how the manager of the master list of evidence is chosen and employed.
55. Discuss the role of the prosecutor in the scene investigation. Is the prosecutor given the power of scene investigation? Or is the scene investigation a police function? How may a prosecutor shape and form a scene investigation?
56. What is the role of the autopsy on the vehicles involved in roadway accidents? Who does the roadway analysis on single-vehicle accidents and where are the results registered and evaluated? Are there certified automotive crash experts? What are some of the precise examinations applicable to liability in automotive accidents (e.g., light filament fracturing)? What is the role of cell phone record examination in automotive scene reconstruction? Review the recent papers on vehicular accidents in the engineering section of the American Academy of Forensic Sciences (AAFS). M

Vocabulary

Automotive safety engineer
Boundaries and margins
Craniocerebral injuries
Crushing injuries to the head and torso
Department of Transportation (state and federal)
Department of Transportation health examinations
Engineering standards
Federal roadway safety guidelines
Guard and protect
Identify and classify
Incapacitated drivers and pilots
Isolation and evaluation

Metal crystallization and failure
Monitor and maintain
Multiple traumatic injuries
Open fracture
Ten-point identification
Traumatic asphyxia
Traumatic exsanguinations
X-ray analysis of metals

Bibliography

Books and Articles

Finkbeiner, W. E., Ursell, P. C., and Davis, R. L. *Autopsy Pathology: A Manual and Atlas*. 2nd ed. St. Louis, MO: Elsevier, 2009.
Stocker, J. T., Dehner, L. P., and Husain, A. N. *Stocker & Dehner's Pediatric Pathology*. 3rd ed. Philadelphia: Lippincott Williams & Wilkins, 2011.
Warrington, D. Marking evidence at crime scenes: Developing a system. *Forensic Magazine* 6, no. 1 (2009): 31–32.

Periodical

Evidence Technology Magazine, www.evidencemagazine.com

Other Resources

Saint Louis University has presented a scene investigation course for years started by George Gantner, MD. Its Web site, www.slu.edu, will provide valuable details on scene investigation and the scene curriculum. Mary Fran Ernst, BLS, the director of this program, became the president of the American Academy of Forensic Sciences in 2002. This program is highly recommended especially to beginners.

A company claiming to have the widest selection of crime scene investigation products is Forensics Source (www.forensicssource.com), which, along with others, advertises in *Forensic Magazine* (www.forensicmag.com). A quick and easy way to stay up-to-date in forensic tools is attendance at the AAFS meeting displays.

Identification: Problems and Methods 7

The great unsolved problem of the forensic sciences was "who?" Although fingerprints were a reliable technique, there were problems. All was solved by Alec Jeffries's 1985 discovery in England of the variable electrophoretic patterns of cellular fragmented DNA. His work was patented by British Biochemical. He reported his findings in the journal *Nature* and some of his first demonstrations of the precision of this technique were solutions to forensic problems of parenthood and relationships. Small world.

Objectives

1. Discuss and compare the differences and relationship of police identification to medical examiner identification. M
2. Indicate the problems that arise between dual identification by both medical examiner and police authority; compare with jurisdictions with only one source of identification. M
3. List the descriptive terms and data used by police in their identification. M
4. Who was Alphonse Bertillon? What is the Bertillon method? M
5. What is anthropometry? M
6. What is the Henry method of fingerprint identification and who was Edward R. Henry? What was his major contribution to the science of fingerprinting?
7. Describe the automated fingerprint retrieval system. Discuss the role of the FBI in the development and maintenance of fingerprint identification methods. M
8. Discuss the use of scars and other body deformities—including fractures, occupational body reactions, tattoos, teeth marks, eye patterns, retinal patterns, and dental structures and changes—in the task of personal identification. M
9. Name the age-dependent morphological characteristics of the following age groups: newborn, premature, 2-year-old infant, 8-year-old girl, 16-year-old child, 36-year-old male or female, 54-year-old male or female, and an 86-year-old male or female. S
10. What is the current role of defined centers of ossification in the estimation of the age of a skeleton or group of bones? M

11. Name three non-FBI bone specialists you could call for consultation in a typical osteology case. S
12. Name an association and group from which physical anthropologists may be contracted to perform forensic identifications. S
13. What is meant by Pearson's formula for reconstruction of living stature from femur size? M
14. Describe three cases in which reconstruction of the body or body parts have to be conducive to the solution of the case. M
15. Identify the major fibers available for examination in American forensic pathology. S
16. Describe the differences in human hair according to: M
    Sex
    Race
    Age
    Hair dying
    Chemical-induced change
    Temperature-induced change
17. Identify representative specimens of fibers by microscopy: S
    Vegetable
    Hair
    Plastic
    Plastic rug
    Cotton towel
    Collagen
18. Describe the methods usually used in identification under the following circumstances:
    Body without hands
    Body presenting as "charred remains"
    Disarticulated body found at various scenes and times
    Body in which the traumatic injuries have made facial identification unreliable or impossible
    Decomposing body with intact clothing
    Decomposing body with tattoos, intact teeth, intact scalp hair, nondecomposed fingers and fingertips, and recent stomach contents
    Unidentified body with measurable femur length
    Body with intact upper and lower dental plates
19. What are the minimal standards of identification that are acceptable in a medical examiner's day-to-day working situation? With infants, is parental identification alone satisfactory? Under what circumstances? M
20. Discuss the development of composite drawing techniques used by police agencies in identifications. M

21. Discuss the role of identification problems when part of the missing person problem. Discuss the problem of identification in regard to the holding of bodies until identified. What is the logical or appropriate time for holding and what standards are met to reach an appropriate identification? M
22. Discuss the problem of delay in the submission and return of finger-print identifications to local, state, and federal agencies. M

Dental Forensics

23. What are the guidelines on the use of dental forensic expertise? When is the specialist called in? M
24. Describe the methods used in the description of the dental arcades and their contents. M
25. Describe the use of forensic odontology in identification problems. M
26. How did the application of DNA skin swabs affect the use of forensic odontological bite-mark evidence? M
27. Describe the current methods of tooth imprint and bite analysis.
28. Describe the usual flow of information in a missing persons case. Start at the initial report of the caregiver to the final presumption of loss of identity. Discuss the care of skeletal remains, decomposing and putrefying remains, and fresh specimens with and without rigor of the masseter muscles. M
29. How are the "number of points of identity" used in identification systems? What are the limits? M
30. Describe the problems that arise with visual identification of bodies at medical examiner/coroner offices. M
31. Describe the use of remote cameras and television systems in identification systems. M
32. Describe the use of Polaroid and cell phone cameras in rapid identification systems. M
33. Discuss the means by which an unidentified body is certified as to the cause of death and how the list of identifying characteristics of the body and scene is established. M
34. The time taken to analyze for DNA as an unknown in a typical real-world case is measured as over fifty hours by some DNA analysts. Can you comment? M

Vocabulary

Bite-mark evidence
Cranial suture identification

Dactylography
Dental casts
Hair, fibers, nail scrapings
Identification by callosities
Identification by teeth marks
Pubic symphysis age changes
Resurrectionists
Teeth marks

Bibliography

Books and Articles

Adelson, L. *The Pathology of Homicide.* Springfield, IL: C.C. Thomas, Springfield, IL, 1974, pp. 1-976. PreDNA identification is covered in the identification section of the very valuable text by Lester Adelson MD, who covered Cleveland Ohio coroner's office pathology in the 40s, 50s, and 60s. His book includes mode, manner and cause of death, the declaring of homicide by the pathologist, autopsy methodology, homicide as crime, justice, and excused behavior, mishandling evidence, scene visits and identification, the clock and calendar of homicide, firearms, cutting, blunt violence, cervical compression, drowning, fire homicide, rape and sexual murder, criminal abortion, poisoning, unusual cases, alcoholism, and the pathologist as a witness. This is a classic text and should be read.

Butler, J. M. *Forensic DNA Typing: Biology, Technology, and Genetics of STR Markers.* 2nd ed. Boston: Elsevier, 2005; several editions. A classic.

Li, R. *Forensic Biology: Identification and DNA Analysis of Biological Evidence.* Boca Raton, FL: CRC Press, 2008; 430 pages.

Sargent, H. R. DNA in the real world. *Evidence Technology Magazine*, April 2007, pp. 12–36.

Silver, W. E., and Souviron, R. R. *Dental Autopsy.* Boca Raton, FL: CRC Press, 2009. The authors both work in the Miami medical examiner's office.

Guidelines and Training Courses

Principles of Forensic DNA for Officers of the Court. Available at www.dna.gov/training/otc. An online version is free of charge at www.dna.gov/training/otc. A cd-rom version is available free with a request of publication number NCH 212399 (there will be a shipping fee).

What Every Law Enforcement Officer Should Know about DNA Evidence. Available at www.dna.gov/training. There is a beginning and an advanced module available.

Organization

Chromosomal Laboratories Inc., 1825 W. Crest Lane, Phoenix, AZ 66027. www.
chromosomal-labs.com. Chromosomal Laboratories is a analytical laboratory
specializing in DNA analysis for forensic casework. *The ChromoZone Forensic
News,* a quarterly newsletter.

Other Resources

A recent film from the Los Angeles, California coroner's office is available describing
their handling of over a thousand problem unclaimed bodies a year See your
local public library.

National Violent Death Reporting System has data used in the journal *Injury
Prevention*; a free supplement is available at the http://ip.bmj.com/

Reliagene Technologies, Inc. New Orleans, LA. Nuclear STR testing ($995). This
group really moves. Y chromosome STR testing ($1275); mitochondrial DNA
($1995); expert witness $200/hour consultation/review; Y STR products; Y-Plex
12 $1000 kit. 1-800-paternity; www.reliagene.com, J.S. Tabak.

There is an American Society for Identification available on the Internet. The specialty boards for the various forensic specialty groups are listed under "reference" in the annual AAFS directory. Identification, photography, forensic art,
and several other disciplines are bunched into the general section until they are
large and strong enough to merit a separate section. Obviously, the switch to a
dominance by the criminalistics section is related to the economic changes in
forensic science.

Postmortem Changes (Signs of Death)

8

Objectives

1. Dead bodies are described in morgue jargon (slang) by their appearances and conditions. These terms are for quick, convenient communication and are not meant for the ears of the uninitiated. Be tactful.
   Stinker
   Floater
   Jumper
   Whale or land whale
   Bone
   Mummy
   Junkie
   Transvestite or he-she
   Traffic
   Crib death, baby death
   Cooked, fried, charred
   Hanger
   Close contact
   Head case

2. Discuss the Harvard criteria for the phenomenon of cerebral death. What are some of the confounding circumstances of heart–lung death? Describe the proper method for heart tone and respiration sound detection. Describe the proper way to check the corneal reflexes. Describe a reliable examination to demonstrate the absence of brain stem function. How is the EEG used in the determination of brain death? What considerations for oxygenation are taken in cases of organ donation? How is cerebral blood flow distinguished? M, S

3. Discuss the interrelationship of the vital medullary centers, the lungs function, the cardiac function, and the flow of blood in the loss (extinction) of life as is commonly experienced in public death. M

4. In a linear order of time, discuss the early postmortem changes up to the time period of six hours. M

5. Discuss some of the unique terminal physiological changes seen in the death of an organism. Include ejaculation and terminal peristalsis. What is purging? M

6. Discuss the evidentiary value of the chemical changes seen in the vitreous humor of dying people. Describe the work of John Coe, MD, in this area. M

7. Discuss the early chemistry of death as indicated by various body fluids: blood, cerebrospinal fluid, and vitreous humor. M

8. What is meant by postmortem lividity? Discuss its pathophysiology. M

9. Discuss the pathophysiology of rigor mortis. M

10. Discuss the Anglo-Saxon rules of the onset of death with cessation of heartbeat and respiration. M

11. Discuss the phenomenon of the loss of body heat with death. M

12. Describe the usual methods for the determination of the time of death in urban public deaths. M

13. What precautions are made about the time of death when testifying in a court proceeding? M

14. What is putrefaction and what are its mechanisms?

15. Describe the process of mummification of a dead human body. M

16. When and where is the process of mummification part of the postmortem change in American forensic pathology? M

17. What is the biochemical change seen in adipocere formation? M

18. Discuss the changes seen in bodies exposed to these circumstances: M
    Depressurization of an aircraft
    Depressurization of a submarine craft
    Extreme heat exposure as a flash or over a time period
    Extreme cold exposure

19. Discuss postmortem coloration in relationship to the following: M
    Reduced hemoglobin
    Carboxyhemoglobin
    Cyanohemoglobin
    Methemoglobin

20. What is cutis anserina? Discuss its origin and postmortem appearance. M

21. What is meant by cadaveric spasm related to instantaneous rigor mortis? M

22. What is putrefactive hemolysis and when does it occur? M

23. Describe the actions of gas-forming bacteria in postmortem situations. M

24. Why should a body decompose rapidly with associated gas formation and discoloration in the tissues of the body? M

25. What are the natural limits to the advancing speed of decomposition? M

26. How does one culture the offending septicemic organism when it is a gas forming *Clostridium perfringens (C. welchii)*? M
27. Discuss the role of various room environments with the development of postmortem autolysis. M
28. Discuss the breakdown of hemoglobin and relate it to the various pigments seen in decomposition. M
29. What is anthropophagic activity and under what circumstances might it occur? M
30. Discuss the changes seen in the body after a heavy (hard) and a light (soft) embalming. M
31. Give a time of decomposition for an embalmed or otherwise preserved body. What is the most common mechanism for decay in the embalmed body? M
32. Discuss the evidentiary nature of bodies that have been cremated. M
33. By what means may the postmortem interval be defined? Be complete in your analysis. M
34. Discuss and describe the postmortem changes seen in the following organ systems: hair, skin, eyeballs, oral cavity, naval, genitalia, anus, hands, and feet. M
35. Discuss the management of a discovered body that has been frozen solid and needs an autopsy. M
36. In what circumstances may the postmortem condition of the body be a hazard to the health of the prosector or the environment. M
37. Name several anatomical areas of the body that need special postmortem dissections for evaluation of pertinent or unusual pathological processes. M
38. Describe the dissection and pathological study of the eyes in cases of shaken baby syndrome. Discuss the use of the vitreous humor in the investigation of the postvaccine reaction phenomenon. M
39. Describe the limitations of immunohistochemistry secondary to postmortem decomposition. What is meant by the expression a "stale body" and what is its significance? M
40. Know the instructions given by the Centers for Disease Control and Prevention for completing the cause-of-death section of the death certificate (www.cdc.gov).

Vocabulary

Absent corneal reflexes
Absent papillary response
Adipocere formation
Algor mortis

Biological forensic indicators (e.g., beetles)
Bloat
Blood stain pattern analysis
Body fluids and waste products
Botanical transfer and positional indicators
Cause of death statement
Cleanup and disposal
Decay and its properties
Decomposition
Dehydration and autolysis
Desquamation
Discoloration and foul smell
Disintegration
Exudates and skin blisters
Fatal agent (pathological/etiological agent)
Fatal derangement (pathological process)
Heart–lung death
Hemoglobin reduction
Immediate cause of death (line *a* on death certificate)
Iris reactivity
Livor and lividity; livor mortis
Manner, mechanism, mode of death
Molecular pathology
Nonspecific anatomical process (structural)
Nonspecific physiological process (functional)
Palliation with and without narcotics
Periprocedural death
Profound coma and brain death
Purge and purging
Putrefaction
Putrefaction and purging
Putrid
Qualified cause of death statement
Qualifying—probable, presumed, unknown, unspecified, undetermined, unwitnessed, unrecorded, uncertain
Radionuclide tracer
Retinal boxcar red cells
Rigor mortis and loss of ATP
Risk factors—medical, behavioral, environmental, demographic
Sanitation
Specific condition and specific paradox (incorrect citation)
Split format of certification—duplications of statements
Steam cleaning

Superficial venous patterns
Surface anatomy and pathology
Swelling and gaseous decomposition
Taches noires and global softening
Terminal event/mechanistic terminal event
Time since death indicators
Vitreous potassium
Wound interpretation

Bibliography

The College of American Pathologists (www.cap.org) has a number of publications worth reviewing:

Aiding the Living by Understanding Death [Brochure]
Autopsy Performance and Reporting, 2nd ed.
CAP Handbook for the Postmortem Identification of Unidentified Remains, 2nd ed.
Cause of Death and Death Certification: Important Information for Physicians, Coroners, Medical Examiners, and the Public, edited by R. Hanzlick, 2006.
Handbook of Forensic Pathology, 2nd ed.
The Pathologist in Court

The Medical Legal Autopsy and the Ethics of Pathological Diagnosis by Forensic Pathologists; Suicide as a Topic Area in Forensic Pathology

9

Suicide is presented with ethics because it is still a very troublesome event in the human condition. Many services are modern and elite until their management of suicide is evaluated. The standards should be well established in the law and its management should be monitored by the attorney general's office.

Objectives

1. Know the performance of the routine hospital autopsy following the methods of Virchow and Rokitansky following selective vascular dissection, including posterior and lateral neck, brain stem, skull base, middle and inner ears, sphenoid fossa, pituitary, anterior ethmoid, cervical vertebrae, cardiac, lung, esophageal, and pelvic areas.
2. Understand use of the Stryker saw or similar vibrating saw, blade replacement, tool sharpening, scales, probes, scissors, knives, and body lifts. S
3. Demonstrate toxicology specimen collection with proper containers and prompt delivery to toxicology with proper techniques (sealed and dated containers with chain of custody). S
4. Demonstrate biological specimen collection, including serology and DNA. S
5. Understand trace evidence and nonroutine evidence handling. S
6. Describe subdural hematoma collection and analysis. S
7. Describe techniques for electron, digital, comparative, and special microscopy. S
8. Know rape examination with vital and nonvital cytological examination. S
9. Discuss spinal cord removal with vertebral column dissection anterior and posterior neck dissections. S
10. Understand air embolism detection and collection technology. S
11. Describe trace metal analysis methodology. S

69

12. Discuss environmental autopsy techniques. S
13. Describe special scenes analysis with suicide risk assessment and potential scale formulation. S
14. Discuss the problem of consent for medicolegal autopsies and indicate its various interpretations including in Alabama, California, Maryland, and New York. M
15. Under what conditions is a forensic pathologist responsible for a complete autopsy, incomplete autopsy, and nonperformance of an autopsy? M
16. List the proper equipment and tools and environmental conditioning necessary for a modern autopsy room. Make a list of the autopsy equipment that can be purchased at local retailers. M
17. Provide a flow diagram for a body (cadaver) movement from the scene to the autopsy theater to the storage cooler in idealized conditions. M
18. Discuss the relationship of the forensic autopsy room to the embalming process and body storage. Describe the relationships with cremation and ash disposal. M
19. Discuss the proper methods for the measurement and weighing of organs. M
20. Describe the quality control methods for organ weights and sizes. M
21. Discuss the proper utilization of photography in the forensic autopsy. Give an outline of the descriptive techniques of the forensic autopsy. Define descriptive morphology. M
22. Describe a method for the description of one to multiple (25) gunshot wounds to the body. What is your preferred reference site for vertical and horizontal measurement? Explain. What is your method for body handling during the measuring of the bullet wounds? What precautions do you take to avoid losing a loose bullet? How do you use a long metal bullet probe in gunshot wound cases? What are the precautions with its use? How do you retrieve a subcutaneous palpable bullet pellet? And how do you handle it as evidence? If a bullet pellet is found loose in the body bag, how do you identify it and retain it for the ballistics lab? Do you describe, excise, and preserve each entry/exit wound? Why? How do you store them? Describe the different skin changes (inshoot and outshoot) as they relate to the velocity and caliber of the bullet. Do you x-ray every shooting case? What is your policy in this matter? What is your preferred method of gunshot wound description in the autopsy protocol?
23. Describe the autopsy methodology with special techniques in the following conditions: M, S
     Acute pulmonary tuberculosis
     Acute heavy metal poisoning

Acute viral pneumonitis

Acute and chronic aspiration pneumonitis

Viral, bacterial, fungal, and parasitic meningitis

Crib death and faulty crib construction death

Acute myocardial infarction

Geriatric arteriosclerosis

Congenital cardiovascular disease

Acute appendicitis and diffuse peritonitis

Acute perforated peptic ulcer

Aplenic rupture with/without trauma

24. Describe the proper method for the opening of a skull in the instance of closed head injury. What tools would you use and what imaging techniques are called for? M, S

25. Describe the anterior and posterior approaches to cervical traumatic lesions. M, S

26. Identify the methods of spinal cord injury demonstration. M, S

27. Identify the methods used to demonstrate the origin of pulmonary emboli. M, S

28. Demonstrate the autopsy methods for the determination of the site of origin of pulmonary emboli. S

29. Discuss the problem of fat embolization and its demonstration in the autopsy. M, S

30. Describe the methods of bacterial culturing in forensic cases. M, S

31. Demonstrate the appropriate method for drawing a clean sterile and adequate blood culture in a morgue or crime scene site. S

32. Describe methods and special techniques used in the examination of exhumed bodies. M, S

33. Indicate the rationale for the following techniques: M

Limited or partial autopsy

Inspections

Full autopsy with toxicology

Full autopsy without toxicology but with neuropathology

Special organ autopsy

Procedural related autopsy

34. In what circumstance can the opening of the large and small intestine be passed over and omitted from the routine? What technical concerns are there in the opening of the bowels? How are stomach contents described and retained? When are stomach contents sent to toxicology? What is the glass funnel technique of stomach content assessment? What specific drug container is found in stomach contents? How is methadone packaged for use in the treatment of long-term cancer pain therapy? M

35. What is the rationale for the examination or nonexamination of the spinal cord in some autopsies? M
36. Discuss the second autopsy and its professional and scientific implications. M
37. What are the conditions in which second autopsies are usually performed? M
38. Discuss the role of the dictation of the autopsy protocol utilizing the following enumerated techniques: M, S
    Computerized descriptive autopsy technique
    Prescribed autopsy format technique (boilerplate)
    Positive lesion identification technique
    Data management technique (i.e., access)
39. Discuss the use of the following autopsy table techniques: M, S
    In situ movie cameras and projectors
    In situ dictation equipment
    Stationary video camera systems
40. Discuss the relative merits of the complete descriptive autopsy format as compared with the positive findings autopsy format. M
41. Discuss the secretarial workload in an autopsy service and its relationships to the work and efficiency of the forensic pathologist. Discuss the current morgue computerized management systems, their cost, and their utility. What is "autopsy report bankruptcy"? M
42. Discuss how the services of a neuropathologist are integrated into a medical examiner's system. Describe the levels and degrees of service. Delineate the funding and equipping of a neuropathology laboratory. Distinguish a forensic service laboratory from a forensic research laboratory by mission, protocol, and certification. M
43. Describe the technical handling of the body tissues after the autopsy is completed. Include levels of anatomical definition, degrees of disease identification, the use of reference resources, and final disposition of the tissues. M
44. What are the methods of the handling and study of histological specimens after the autopsy is completed? M
45. Discuss the identification methods for tissue sections. What differentiates forensic histology from ordinary histology? What is forensic cytology? What are cell surface markers? M
46. Discuss the various fixatives used in forensic cases. M
47. Discuss the histology workload and the workload recording data systems available for the forensic autopsy. M
48. Discuss the utilization of forensic pathology peers to review autopsy findings. M
49. Discuss quality control issues in forensic pathology and in the forensic autopsy. M

50. List the available references on forensic autopsy techniques. Can you relate the various countries of origin to the texts? M
51. Outline the secretarial paper flow for forensic autopsies. How are the currently used medical record systems for forensic offices providing new epidemiological information? And how is it used in forensic analysis? M, S
52 Enumerate the topic areas where records must be kept in a medico-legal system. M
53. Explain the various techniques used in finalizing a forensic autopsy. M
54. Give examples of "final decisions." M
55. Review medical ethics; see Wikipedia coverage. M
56. Review the ethics of personal and family guidance. M
57. Outline the death registration routine at the county or parish level. S
58. Show how one enables the authority of family representatives. S
59. Show how one enables the authority of religious representatives. What are the potential points of irritation (procedural conflicts) between the pathologist and the undertaker/funeral director? Discuss how these can be controlled and made understandable. M
60. Discuss the responsibility of ensuring proper prosecution of crimes. Where does the concept of stewardship enter into forensic pathology? M
61. What are some sources for key terms and concepts in medical ethics? Is there a text on forensic pathology ethics? Who defines the ethics of forensic pathology? Of pathology? M
62. What are the defining attributes of an expert witness? M
63. Discuss the ethics of revealing personal information in trial testimony. Are witnesses free of ethical responsibility for personal matters? M
64. Discuss the ethics of government inspectors and laboratory quality control as it relates to the special nature of the forensic autopsy and investigation. M
65. What ethical problems may arise between the autopsy pathologist and the prosecutor's examiners and investigators? What is meant by the expression "to make a case." M
66. How is a medical witness protected from malpractice allegations in criminal procedures? In civil procedures? M

Skills

Forensic pathologists should have the following skills applicable at the cause of death autopsy:

Diagnostic frozen sections
Diagnostic cellular smears and imprints

Specific dissections for traumatic and natural processes
Capable forensic photography with immediate review
Case interpretation to expedite the completion of the preliminary
    investigation
Explanation of the psychiatric aspects of the investigation
Careful selection of toxicological, biological, and criminalistic eviden-
    tiary specimens
Appropriate evidence identification and storage
Blue tooth technology with cleared funeral/disposal protocols
Smartphone camera with image transfer
24-hour case report in print and to distribution center
Completed toxicology submission at eight hours
Complete inventory of formalin fixed tissues
Completed preliminaries for brain–nervous system study
Completed requests for supplemental data/studies (OR, ER, EMT)

Vocabulary

Anatomical planes of dissection
Biopsychosocial perspective
Decisions, informed consent, and competence
Statuatory law and informed consent
Withdrawal of treatment and futility
Manners and decorum at the autopsy
Implications from the viewing of the autopsy
Understanding local funeral customs
Rules undertakers and funeral directors follow
Obligations of social and legal character
Duties and responsibilities of the forensic pathologist
Job descriptions for autopsy personnel
Opinions and beliefs: public, private, and political
Biopsychosocial theory
Geriatric pathology and euthanasia
Aging and senescence and advance directives
Body disposition and organ donation
Tolerance to alcohol and pain control
Timing of the physical changes of alcoholism
Consent issues of the autopsy, informed consent
Dissociation and homicide
Moral decision making and ethics consultation

Bibliography

Books

Adelson, L. *The Pathology of Homicide.* Springfield, IL: C.C. Thomas, 1974. An important teaching text based on his autopsy work for the Cuyahoga County Coroners Office (Cleveland, Ohio) at Western Reserve University. It covers the basics of mode, manner and cause of death, identification problems, clock and calendar of homicide investigation, firearms, cuttings, stabbings, blunt violence, cervical compression, chocking, homicide by fire, sex murders, criminal abortion, poisonings in detail, misadventures, unusual homicides, and alcoholism with notes on the pathologist's witness duties.

Autopsy Performance and Reporting. Chicago: CAP Press, 1990.

Baker, R. D. *Postmortem Examination: Specific Methods and Procedures.* Philadelphia: Saunders, 1967.

Burton, J. L., and Rutty, G. N., eds. *The Hospital Autopsy: A Manual of Fundamental Autopsy Practice.* 3rd ed. London: Hodder Arnold, 2010. The text includes the clinical audit, radiology, reconstruction, methods for maternity cases, high risk infections, and anaphylaxis, suite design and construction, external and internal examination, authorization and dissection techniques.

Callahan, D. *What Price Better Health? The Hazards of the Research Imperative.* Berkeley: University of California Press, 2003.

Collins, K. A., and Hutchins, G. M., eds. *Autopsy Performance & Reporting.* 2nd ed. Northfield, IL: College of American Pathologists, 2003.

Finkbeiner, W. E., Ursell, P. C., and Davis, R. L. *Autopsy Pathology: A Manual and Atlas.* 2nd ed. Philadelphia: Saunders, 2010.

Junkerman, C., and Schniedermayer, D. *Practical Ethics for Students, Interns, and Residents: A Short Reference Manual.* 2nd ed. Frederick, MD: University Publishing Group, 1998.

Ludwig, J. *Handbook of Autopsy Practice.* 3rd ed. Totowa, NJ: Humana Press, 2002. A text with good detail.

Organizations

American Association of Suicidology, www.suicidology.org
American Foundation for Suicide Prevention, www.afsp.org
International Association of Forensic Nurses, www.iafn.org
National Institute of Mental Health, www.nimh.nih.gov

Other Resources

Ed Uthman, MD, Houston, Texas, presents his personal system of forensic autopsy free on the Internet. Contact by using the Path-ol list contact.

"Old Red." The University of Texas Medical Branch, one of the oldest surviving medical school buildings west of the Mississippi and one of the few schools on the Gulf Coast, bears a historic lesson in education for all pathologists in the restored Old Red building. This was the original medical school building. It is a semioval room with a strikingly vertical seating arrangement of elevated benches that close in and focus on the central podium. The center is recessed into the floor two steps so there is even more concentration of the view onto the center. This was the place where the instructor would hold the anatomical specimen for all to see. This was the method before photography and loudspeakers. And it worked. This building is open today and is a must-see for all pathologists.

The surgical amphitheater of Children's Hospital, Boston. I watched Robert Gross, MD, chief surgeon of the Boston Children's Hospital, the first surgeon to ligate the neonatal ductus arteriosus, and the early worker/leader on the NIH project on the mechanical heart, perform surgery without his knowing it. I was in the room above his surgical theater, which was separated from him by a large $10^{2\prime}$ 20^2 glass window. I could look down and see his every move. The entire surgical area was visible, even the tables and gear of the surgical nurses and anesthesiologists. It was nothing to spend an hour watching the masters of pediatric surgery at the Children's perform their surgical feats. As a teaching aid there is no other comparable tool. Of course now we have ceiling-mounted TV surveillance cameras that are usually part of a security program, but the glass ceiling approach to surgical observation is unequaled. Since this experience I have always promoted the use of the room above the surgery to be transformed into a surgical teaching area by installation of the ceiling glass window. Autopsy surgery is not an exception.

Suicide Objectives

1. What were Durkheim's four types of suicide?
2. Name some suicide research journals.
3. In the United States where is there a good source of information on suicide?
4. Give a summative statistic on the occurrence of suicide in the United States.
5. Is suicide a preventable disease?
6. The prevalence of treatment of the mentally ill varies with the cultural and political and other associated conditions. Most would agree that a 40% treatment figure applies to most American related suicidal situations. Discuss this from the standpoint of mental health. M
7. Sixty percent of suicide victims have previous (one month) treatment for their psychiatric condition. Discuss and relate to the present status of public health care. M
8. What are the particular problems with a suicide autopsy? Do you expect/anticipate a very close review both by an experienced autopsy pathologist and a suicide specialist from the mental health services (psychiatry or psychology)?

9. Should the coroner/medical examiner autopsy performed be:

    A meticulous dissection and identification of each morphological variable: skin marks, foreign bodies, smells, arterial and venous transactions, organ perforations, and so forth?

    Careful detailed description and sampling of the clothing including socks and shoes?

    Close collaboration with the investigating police authority?

    A fully evaluated list of forensic science applications to be fulfilled in case completion?

    Complete toxicological studies with an associated review of the drug containers at the scene and at home?

    A second review of circumstances with the witness group?

    A multiview photography of the mechanisms of death with reviewed continuity of all devices, ropes, cords, clothing, etc.?

10. How do you manage the anticipated family and work problems when properly recording the cause of death and its circumstances; for example, denying suicide for different purposes (management or political or social)? M

11. In some circumstances an appeal of a lower court judicial opinion of an accident in the case of a bona-fide suicide may require an appeal from the state attorney general's office to a higher court. The continued concern of the pathologist to the case outcome may be definitive in effect. This is not an unusual problem and the proper management of these cases will determine the community evaluation of the forensic services. Comment on these statements. M

12. Remembering the distinction between witnessed events and unwitnessed events, how should the pathologist question the witness? Who is responsible for the careful presentation of the witnesses' statements? M

13. What is meant by the *law of availability* in suicide methodology analysis? Give some examples of how this law works. M

Bibliography

Books and Articles

Durkheim, E. *Suicide: A Study in Sociology.* New York: Free Press, 1951.

Hough, D. and Lewis, P. A. Suicide prevention advisory group at an academic medical center. *Military Medicine* 175, no. 5 (2010): 347–351.

Humphrey, D. *Dying with Dignity: Understanding Euthanasia.* Secaucus, NJ: Carol Publishing Group, 1992.

Leenaars, A. A., Park, B., Collins, P. I., Wenckstern, S., and Leenaars, L. Martyrs' last letters: Are they the same as suicide notes? *Journal of Forensic Science* 55, no. 3 (2010): 660–668.

Schneidman, E. *Comprehending Suicide: Landmarks in Twentieth Century Suicidology.* Washington, DC: American Psychological Association, 2001.

Stoudemire, A. *Clinical Psychiatry for Medical Students.* 3rd ed. Philadelphia: Lippincott, 1998.

Organizations

American Association of Suicidology (AAS), www.suicidology.org

AMSUS: The Society of the Federal Health Agencies, www.amsus.org. AMSUS also publishes the monthly journal *Military Medicine.*

National Institute of Mental Health (NIMH), www.nimh.nih.gov

The Cause and Mechanisms of Death: Natural Death and the Changes of Aging; Geriatric Pathology; and End-of-Life Care, Hospice Care, and Palliative Care

10

Objectives

1. Distinguish between the terms *cause of death* and *mechanisms of death*. M
2. What is meant by the word construction *proximate cause*? M
3. How is proximate cause used in the legal and medical evaluation of the cause of death? M
4. Discuss the formulation of the death certificate and the various logic schemes used in death certification. M
5. Distinguish and give an example of natural death, accidental death, suicidal death, and homicidal death. M
6. Describe the difference between a witnessed death and an unwitnessed death. M
7. What are the criteria determining the performance or nonperformance of an autopsy? M
8. What is meant by *reliable medical information*? M
9. What is the role of insurance claim and civil suits in the performance of an autopsy by a medicolegal authority? M
10. In what way does the autopsy remove speculation and in what way does it encourage the use of the uncertainty principle? M
11. What is meant by a public death? M
12. What is the expected mortality rate within an American population? How is it contrasted between inner city and suburban areas of large metropolitan areas? M
13. Describe the percentage of cases that would be recognized as coroner/medical examiner cases under usual circumstances and indicate what percentage would be homicides and natural deaths. M

14. Indicate the rough percentage of death that would be due to disease of the cardiovascular system, respiratory system, and central nervous system. M
15. Indicate some of the leading causes of sudden unexpected death in the following systems: M
    Circulatory
    Respiratory
    Digestive
    Urinary
    Central nervous system
16. What are the limits or minimal changes seen in occlusive coronary artery disease? M
17. How does the incidence of arteriosclerosis change from the age periods 20, 40, 60, 80, and 100? M
18. Distinguish naturally occurring lesions causing asphyxia, and compare and contrast them with manual asphyxial changes. M
19. Discuss hemorrhage within the air passages and indicate its usual sites of origin. M
20. Delineate the rarer causes of sudden unexpected natural death. Indicate several from each organ system. M
21. Indicate the reasons for the absence of findings in many geriatric autopsies. M
22. List several references for perinatal, obstetric, genetic, and geriatric pathology. M
23. Discuss the normal activity patterns of persons suffering with extensive myocardial infarction. M
24. Discuss the relationship of both chronic and acute alcoholism with myocardial infarction. M
25. Discuss the usual course of events in sudden death from rupture of a large lower aorta aneurysm. Compare the lumbar site disease with the thoracic site disease. M
26. Discuss the nature of death from an acute spontaneous cerebral hemorrhage. M
27. Compare and contrast the acute spontaneous cerebral hemorrhage to an acute traumatic cerebral hemorrhage. M
28. Discuss the occurrence and appearance of staphyloco deaths of the cerebral circulation. M
29. Compare aneurysms originated from trauma, congenital, and infectious etiologies. M
30. Discuss the incidence and nature of sudden death arising from disease of the respiratory system. M
31. Indicate the major causes of bronchopneumonia. M

32. Diseases of the brain and meninges are often responsible for sudden death. Indicate the usual circumstances and anatomical changes seen. M
33. Identify pachymeningitis interna and discuss its usual course. M
34. Discuss the usual death scene in communicable disease deaths and indicate the usual methods for the identification of the etiological agent. M
35. Indicate the usual autopsy findings in cases of sudden death arising from the following: M
    Perforated peptic ulcer
    Acute appendicitis
    Acute pyelonephritis
    Acute bladder distention
    Massive pulmonary embolus
    Anemia
    Sickle cell disease
36. Discuss the circumstances by which a natural childhood disease can mimic an assault or parental beating. M
37. Discuss growth failure and indicate how it can cause mimicry of traumatic disease. M
38. What is meant by death from neglect? M
39. Indicate the pathological findings in infantile acute diarrheal episodes. M
40. Identify thymicolymphaticus and describe the autopsy findings therein. M
41. Compare *palliative care* (any disease stage, comprehensive and throughout an illness, may maintain curative care, provide comfort, ease symptoms) with *hospice care* (dying patients of any age with no maintenance of curative treatment, use of symptom and pain control, six-month prognosis required by Medicare) in terms of case management, cost, services provided, and key differences. M
42. How do you explain the lack of a formally recognized section of geriatric pathology in American pathology? M
43. Name several successful texts relating to geriatric pathology. M
44. Describe some experimental pathology studies applicable to:
    Drowning
    Electrocution
    Exsanguination
    Asphyxia
    Freezing to death
    Starvation and dehydration
    Acute alcoholism
45. Review the conditions for body donation in your jurisdiction.
46. What expenses may be incurred in medical school body donation?

Vocabulary

Case management
Chronic disease management
Durable power of attorney for health care
End-of-life wishes
Hospice care
Informed consent
Living will
Palliative care
Patient needs
Prolong life
Recovery and rehabilitation

Bibliography

Books and Articles

Bancroft, J. D., and Stevens, A. *Theory and Practice of Histological Techniques*. 2nd ed. Edinboro, Scotland: Churchill Livingstone, 1982.

Duckett, S. *The Pathology of the Aging Human Nervous System*. Philadelphia: Lea & Febiger, 1991.

End of life care: Difficult concerns, caring choices. *St. Louis Metropolitan Medicine* 31, no. 5 (2009): 18–24.

Kaufman, D. L. *Injuries and Illnesses in the Elderly*. St. Louis, MO: Mosby, 1997.

Corrigan, G. E., *Geriatric Pathology Gazette*, volume 1, issues 1-19, November-December, 2000-3.

Knight, J. A. *Laboratory Medicine and the Aging Process*. Chicago: American Society of Clinical Pathology, 1996.

Missouri Office of the Attorney General, *Life Choices*. 2009. Available at http://ago.mo.gov/publications/lifechoices/lifechoices.pdf

Organizations

American Academy of Hospice and Palliative Medicine, www.aahpm.org

Missouri Bar Association, www.mobar.org. Sample advance directive forms for effect when the patient is terminal or persistently unconscious.

Missouri End-of-Life Coalition, www.mo-endoflife.org

National Hospice and Palliative Care Organization, with a physician resource center; www.nhpco.org

Sudden Death: Forensic Clinical Microbiology

11

Objectives

1. Distinguish and define the following: M
   Sudden death
   Unexpected death
   Sudden and unexpected death
   Natural death
   Contributory factors to death
   Witnessed death
   Instantaneous death
2. Distinguish and describe the class of medical deaths recognized as "deaths from fright." M
3. Distinguish and describe the medical events in comatose death and describe the varieties of comatose death scenes. M
4. Distinguish and classify deaths that follow trauma and deaths that are posttraumatic but natural in origin. M
5. Discuss the concept of the prediabetic state and discuss the relationship of trauma to the development of the diabetic state. Discuss the role of the Eli Lilly Corporation of Indianapolis, Indiana, in the development of the science of diabetic death. What was their historical role in diabetes? M
6. Discuss the relationship of trauma to the occurrence of carcinoma. Discuss carcinoma in its theoretical relationships to incomplete and aberrant healing. M
7. Relate a list of laboratory specimens suitable for the study or distinction of diabetes mellitus derivable from an autopsy. Be complete as possible. S
8. Discuss the relationship between deaths with collapse and contrast it to collapse with death. How does one distinguish between these two conditions? M
9. Discuss the phenomena of postmortem contusion, laceration, and abrasion. M
10. Discuss the relationship of posttraumatic injury and the metabolic changes brought into play with the trauma. M
11. Discuss the relationship of trauma, the internal milieu, and the collapse of the homeostatic mechanisms. M

12. Discuss the neurological and the vascular, endocrine, electrolyte, and neurohormonal control of the internal milieu. M
13. Discuss the visual and morphological relationships of the timing of injuries and indicate the relative sensitivities of the following study methods: M
    Gross inspection
    Histological examination
    Biochemical analysis
    Electrophysiology
    Histochemistry
    Immunohistochemistry
14. Distinguish between antemortem wounds and postmortem wounds. Describe the usual head injuries from those who die and fall. M
15. Discuss immediate and delayed shock. M
16. Discuss what is meant by disseminated intravascular coagulation and indicate the specific observations and diagnostic tests used in recognizing this change. M
17. Discuss the etiology, course, development, epidemiology, and forensic consequences of crib death (SIDS, sudden unexpected death in infancy, cot death). What is the expected pulmonary pathological change seen in these infants? What is the natural frequency of crib death in the United States? M
18. In the circumstance of an alcoholic mother overlying and suffocating her cosleeping two-month-old infant, what is the consequence of an elevated maternal blood alcohol level? What charge may be made by the prosecutor? What is the role of intent in this type of homicide? M
19. Is the presence of an cosleeping alcoholic mother a source of child endangerment and require separation? Discuss.
20. Discuss the role of the forensic pathologist as a witness in child endangerment cases. M

Note

When I first went to Children's Hospital in Boston, I found that at the autopsies we set up our own bacteriological cultures. None of this "take a swab and send it to the lab." Our swabs went directly into tubes and onto plates kept in the autopsy room incubator. Fresh media was delivered weekly. The day after the autopsy and the necessary days after that, the microbiology tech (a senior tech with a master's degree) came and read the plates with us. Hands on. The answer was delivered as he made the identification right there. Of course, he took the variants back to his lab. Remember he had previously cultured most of our patients. The incubator was a small 3' × 2' box with a central thermometer. The media was kept in the morgue refrigerator. This was direct and simple.

Vocabulary

Abusive head injury
Accidental falls
Accidental positional asphyxia
Adolescent hanging
Airbag sodium azide
Appropriate evidence
Cardiac life support
Cerebral edema
Child abuse
Cosleeping
Database examination
Drowning and asphyxiation
Drug-facilitated crime
Drugs by type, level, legality, number
Exothermic reaction
Forensic epidemiology
Heat-related death
Internal injuries sufficient for death
Laryngotracheobronchitis
Level of investigation
Levels by therapeutic level, lethality, toxicity
Mortality data and vital statistics data
Natural causes
Nerve sheath hemorrhage (NSH)
Nonaccidental injuries
Overlying
Population dynamics and evolution
Postmortem changes
Postmortem perfusion techniques
Prone and supine
Pseudostrangulation
Retinal hemorrhage (RH)
Risky behavior
Substandard investigation
Sudden death
Suffocation

Supervised swimming
TV tip-over infant death
Undetermined cause
Undetermined manner of death

Bibliography

Books and Articles

Donato, S. D., Neri, M., and Maglietta, R. A. Sudden Death from Atypical Pneumonia in a Healthy Adolescent. *Proceedings of the American Academy of Forensic Sciences 62nd Annual Scientific Meeting,* Seattle, WA, 2010.

Garcia, L. S., ed. *Clinical Microbiology Procedures Handbook.* 3rd ed. 3 vols. Washington, DC: ASM Press, 2010.

Koehler, S. A. Forensic epidemiology and the forensic nurse. In *Forensic Nursing Science,* 2nd ed., edited by V. A. Lynch and J. B. Duval, Chapter 4. St. Louis, MO: Mosby, 2011.

Larsen, M. K., Nissen, P. H., Kristensen, I. B., Jensen, H. K., Lundemose, J. B. Genetic Aspects of Sudden Death in Youth: A Retrospective Study of Familial Hypercholesterolemia. *Proceedings of the American Academy of Forensic Sciences 62nd Annual Scientific Meeting,* Seattle, WA, 2010.

Maulean, G., Tabib, A., Malicier, D., and Fanton, L. Sudden Death Due to Mesothelioma of the Atrio-Ventricular Node. *Proceedings of the American Academy of Forensic Sciences 62nd Annual Scientific Meeting,* Seattle, WA, 2010.

Meyers, W. M., ed. *Pathology of Infectious Diseases.* Vol. 1, *The Helminthiases.* Washington, DC: American Registry of Pathology, 2000.

Murray, P. R., Barron, E. J., Jorgensen, J. H., Landry, M. L., and Pfaller, M. A. *Manual of Clinical Microbiology.* 9th ed. 2 vols. Washington, DC: ASM Press, 2007. A bench companion and a media book are among other publications.

Saint-Martin, P., Byrne, P. O., Gaulier, J. M., and Dupont, S. M. Undiagnosed, Untreated Acute Promyelocytic Leukemia Presenting as Suspicious. *Proceedings of the American Academy of Forensic Sciences 62nd Annual Scientific Meeting,* Seattle, WA, 2010.

Stevens, S. *Forensic Nurse: The New Role of the Nurse in Law Enforcement.* New York: Thomas Dunne, 2004.

Woods, G. L., Gutierrez, Y., Walker, D., Purtilo, D. T., and Stanley, J. D. *Diagnostic Pathology of Infectious Diseases.* Philadelphia: Lea & Febiger, 1993.

Organizations

American Association of Clinical Chemistry, www.AACC.org
American Society for Microbiology, www.asm.org
Hardy Diagnostics, 1430 West McCoy Lane, Santa Maria, CA 93456. www.hardydiagnostics.com. A complete lab service with extensive e-mail and supply catalog service in all aspects of microbiology and parasitology. Direct mail service with latest updates. Questions answered by their customer service and tech service departments.

Physical Trauma

12

Objectives

1. Briefly describe the changes in each of the following trauma classifications. M
   - Blunt physical trauma
   - Sharp physical trauma
   - Sharp penetrating trauma
   - Physical trauma with local penetration

   Describe how they are altered by immediate and prolonged immersion in a fresh water lake. M
2. Give several examples of each of the above described physical trauma types. M
3. Describe the histological tissue changes seen in blunt physical trauma. M
4. Describe the findings of massive body contusions as seen in the London air raid bombings of 1942. What syndrome evolved from these studies? M
5. Describe the typical traumatic changes of the head and the face of passengers in automobile accidents. M
6. Describe the usual or typical traumatic changes in a "jumper." What ancillary studies are carried out in these cases? M
7. Describe the physical trauma in the cases of forcible mechanical lethal body compression. Distinguish the relative elastic coefficients of various portions and tissues of the body. M
8. Distinguish the external changes seen in heat injury as follows M
   - Hot wet heat
   - Hot dry heat
   - High velocity dry heat
9. Present the histological findings seen in heat injury. Discuss the changes in the blood in hot heat injury. M
10. Discuss the traumatic lesions seen in frostbite. Distinguish them from heat injury. M
11. Describe the physical findings seen in freezing injury. Delineate the differences from frostbite. M

12. Discuss the superficial changes seen in cold injury to the skin. M
13. Distinguish the injuries to the skin seen in basic solution burns, as in lye. What are the major histological changes of lye burns? M
14. Distinguish the external features of acid burns. Delineate the histological changes seen in acid burns. M
15. Describe the internal gastrointestinal changes seen in acid and lye burns. Are there latent or delayed changes seen in these injuries? How are they treated? M
16. How may radiation death be distinguished at a gross and microscopic level? What are the external changes of radiation injury? M
17. Enumerate the changes seen in the Hiroshima bomb victims. Distinguish the acute, subacute, and chronic changes. M
18. What is radiation fibroblast and what is its meaning? M
19. Discuss the utility of the radiation detector badge among those who work with radiation or radiation problems. M
20. Discuss the following sources of trauma: M
    Light radiation
    Laser beam
    Ultraviolet light
    Magnetic waves with projections
    Long wave radiation
    Radar radiation
    Beer bottle to the head
    Ball-peen hammer to the head
    Flashlight (burglar type) to the head
    Small crowbar (burglar type)
    Tightened fist in the abdomen
    Pointed toe in the ribs
    Knee in the gut or in the testes
21. What is the electromagnetic spectrum and how are its elements detected? M
22. Distinguish the monitoring of analytical equipment utilizable in the study of traumatic injury:
    Chemical
    Thermal
    Electric
    Physical
    Radiation
23. What is a hardness tester? What is a micrometer? M
24. Describe the histological effects of sound waves. M
25. Does wearing a helmet while riding a bike or driving a car provide any benefit to one's safety? M

Vocabulary

Abrasion and road rash
Beta-amyloid precursor protein
Contusion
Fracture
Incomplete skeletal recovery
Laceration
Patterned injury
Repeated stress injury
Schmorl's nodes
Skeletal rapid loading events
Vertebral nucleus pulposus herniation

Bibliography

Mothers Against Drunk Driving, www.madd.org; 511 E. John Carpenter Freeway, Suite 700, Irving, Texas 75062; 1-800-GET-MADD.

Secondary Effects and Complications of Trauma

13

Objectives

1. Describe the usual biochemical changes seen in a simple spiral fracture of distal tibia. M
2. Describe the healing stages of a bone fracture and indicate the clinical enzymology of its healing. M
3. Describe the phenomena of embolization. Enumerate the various types of emboli and discuss their frequency. M
4. Describe the usual and some unusual circumstances of fat emboli. M
5. Describe the phenomena of the migrating bullet. M
6. Define a pathological fracture and indicate the problems that might arise from its occurrence. M
7. Describe the acute and chronic effects of complications of a blunt injury to the skull. M
8. Describe the chronic conditions arising from cervical spine trauma. M
9. Describe the acute and chronic conditions arising from compressive injuries to the chest. M
10. Describe the usual sites of laceration and tear in blunt abdominal trauma, in vehicular crashes, and in school bus accidents. M
11. Describe the changes seen in renal function when there is blunt trauma to the urinary system. M
12. Describe the changes seen in the urinary bladder with various degrees of compressive force. M
13. Describe avulsion injury to the genitalia and indicate the circumstances in which it generally arises. M
14. Describe the changes seen in crushing injuries to the extremities. Indicate significant laboratory findings in these cases. M
15. Describe the diagnostic complications seen in the spinal cord injury patient. M
16. Define shock and indicate its relationship to the functioning of the vascular system. M
17. Describe the injury-related infections that usually occur after traumatic injury. M

18. What is the usual pattern of hemorrhage seen in trauma to the following regions: M
    Head
    Thorax
    Abdomen
    Extremities
19. Describe the gross central nervous system changes seen in fat embolization. M
20. Discuss fatal systemic air embolism. M
21. Discuss the problems in the treatment and diagnosis of pulmonary embolism following venous thrombosis. M
22. Describe the psychological complications of trauma. Give a classification applicable to these phenomenon. M

Transportation Pathology by Vehicle and by Injury

23. Compare rolled over trucks with rolled over cars. What injuries are looked for in school bus and transportation bus accidents? Discuss the use of changed seat positions and arrangements in traffic fatality reduction programs.
24. Where (type of accident) would the wearing of helmets save the most lives in vehicular trauma?
25. What is the role of the department of transportation in the shame and blame of the motor vehicle accident epidemic?
26. What is the relative cost of a shoulder on the side of a road? What is the appropriate size for a road shoulder?
27. What are the dangers of automobile airbags? How are injuries from airbags described? Describe the penetrating injuries derived from airbags and explain their occurrence.
28. Discuss the recent use of beta-amyloid precursor protein (BAPP) immunohistochemical staining in the interpretation of pediatric head trauma cases. M

Vocabulary

Automatic weapon recoil and round selection
Beta-amyloid precursor protein staining (BAPP)
Central nervous system
Crushing injuries
Embolism by type and place and duration
Histological multifocal staining
Inconsistency and improbability

Legal limits of intoxication
Logistic regression analysis
Oil Red O
Pediatric death scene enactment
Peripheral nervous system
Postmortem computed tomography
Reaction without premeditation
Retinal hemorrhages
Spontaneous impulsive behavior

Bibliography

Becker, R. O., and Selden, G. *The Body Electric: Electromagnetism and the Foundation of Life*. New York: Morrow Press, 1985.

Franck, H., and Franck, D. *Mathematical Methods for Accident Reconstruction: A Forensic Engineering Perspective*. Boca Raton, FL: CRC Press, 2009. Automotive specifications, momemtum, impact speed, accident reconstruction, mathematics, computer modeling, photogramometry, use of mathematics in reconstruction.

Kimmerle, E. H., and Baraybar, J. P. *Skeletal Trauma: Identification of Injuries Resulting from Human Rights Abuses and Armed Conflict*. New York: CRC Press 2008.

Gunshot Wounds

14

Objectives

1. Describe the use of the word *epidemic* as related to handgun homicide in the United States. M
2. Draw and label the parts of a Saturday night special. Indicate the unique qualities of these guns. M, S
3. Distinguish the expertise of the forensic pathologist and contrast his role in crime investigation with that of the ballistics expert. Distinguish *accuracy* and *precision* in the use of firearms and distinguishing their effects on the body. M
4. Describe the proper handling of a shooter in a homicide from the forensic evidence viewpoint. Include the spectroscopic examination of the shooter's hands and clothing. M
5. Indicate the relationship of the height of entry of a gunshot wound with the height of the shooter. How fast can someone turn his or her body when being shot at? Discuss this. M
6. Describe the proper examination of the clothing in both shooters and victims. M
7. Discuss the question as to whether every shooting victim (dead or alive) should undergo x-ray examination. M
8. Discuss the relevance of lateral body views by x-ray in the study of gunshot wounding. M
9. Compare and contrast low, medium, and high velocity gunshot wounds of the chest and the abdomen. M
10. Compare and contrast low, medium, and high velocity gunshot wounds of the head. M
11. Compare and contrast the inshoot and outshoot wounds of the following weapons: M
    Saturday night special
    High velocity deer rifle
    Shotgun loaded with a deer slug
    Shotgun with a load of buckshot pellets
    Police .38
    Colt 45

Machine gun

AK-47

Carbine

Military rifle

12. Discuss the following phenomenon in gunshot wounds: M

Double entry of two pellets

Tangential entry of a pellet

Double exit of two pellets

Tandem bullet pellets

Bullet emboli

Fragmented bullet pellets

Shattering bullet pellets

Ricochet bullet pellets

13. Discuss the mechanics of the bullet pellet in regard to the following: M

Speed

Torque

Heat

Turbulent path with pellet tumbling

14. Discuss methods of bullet pellet search and include the utilization of various probes. M

15. Trace the proper identification methodology and flow of evidence from the recovery of a bullet pellet from a homicide victim to its presentation in court. M

16. Enumerate the specific areas in postmortem ballistics where misidentification or criminal interference can intervene. M

17. Discuss the utilization of evidence from assassination victims (e.g., Kennedy, King) in the final analysis of the crime and the crime scene. M

18. Compare and contrast the forensic analysis of the assassination of President John Kennedy with the assassination of presidential candidate Robert Kennedy. M

19. Discuss the utilization of the forensic pathologist in the analysis of gunshot wounds of skeletonized bodies. M

20. Discuss the legal privileges of the living patient with a bullet pellet in his or her body. M

21. What is the reason for the removal of all bullet pellets from all dead bodies? M

22. Distinguish between a witnessed shooting and an unwitnessed shooting. M

23. What percentage of shootings involves the police force? Is there a reason for having a nonpolice ballistic expert available in the community? M

24. Compare and contrast the traumatic disruption of tissues and hemorrhage from a direct penetration of a bullet pellet through an organ

and indirect consequences by the associated physical indirect tissue destruction from "concussion waves." Relate this to the changes seen with some spinal cord injuries. M

25. Discuss the forensic consequences of the gas production occurring in the firing of a bullet. Relate this to the changes of close-contact wounding. M

26. Discuss the analysis of the gases from tissues in gunshot wounds and demonstrate their utility. M

27. What proportion of gunshot wound victims have a delayed homicidal death? What specific forensic problems are generally involved in these deaths? M

28. Discuss the proper death certificate phraseology to be utilized with gunshot wound victims. M

29. Describe the usual physical findings seen in a suicidal contact wound of the temple. M

30. Discuss the relationship of the gun cleaning paraphernalia in a suicide case to the intention of the victim. M

31. Distinguish between a revolver and an automatic. Describe their differences in the production of ballistic evidence at a crime scene. M

32. What is black gunpowder? Compare it to other gunpowders. M

33. Draw and label the parts of a bullet cartridge. Indicate the function of each part. M, S

34. Compare and contrast contact, near contact, and distant entry wounds. M

35. What are the ballistic possibilities in the following sets of wounds? M
    Two entrance wounds and one exit wound
    One entrance wound and two exit wounds
    Two entrance wounds and two exit wounds
    Three entrance wounds and two exit wounds

36. What would be the complete range of possibilities for the above sets of wounds? M

37. What is meant by a wound over a supported structure? Compare and contrast wounds when there is support to the underlying tissues. M

38. Discuss how gunshot wounds can be concealed naturally and by malicious intent. M

39. Discuss the circumstances under which there are self-inflicted gunshot wounds with multiple entry sites. M

40. Discuss the proper ballistic handling of a fragmented bullet wound case. M

41. In gunshot wounds of the heart, how can one explain extensive physical activity after the gunshot wound of the heart in which the autopsy reveals a perforation of the ventricular wall? M

42. Discuss the pathophysiology of cardiac tamponade in gunshot wound cases. M
43. Discuss the typical autopsy findings in the case where the bullet pellet passes through a lung. M
44. Discuss a typical autopsy finding of a shotgun wound where the liver is penetrated. M
45. Discuss the topographical relationships of entry wounds when they are scattered over the body or concentrated in a vital region of entry. M
46. Compare and contrast the following: M
    Metallic bomb explosion wounds
    Plastic bomb explosion wound
    Hand grenade shrapnel wound
47. Discuss the changes seen in cases of hydraulic concussion. M
48. Discuss the constant influx of new guns and ammunition into the criminal market and how that affects ballistics expertise. M

Vocabulary

Abrasion collar
Abrasion margin
Automatic gun, pistol
Bifurcation
Bullet burn
Bullet pellet and cartridge case
Burp gun
Cartridge markings
Collateral damage
Colt 45
Derringer pistol
Double entry; double exit
Fabric holes and perforations
Fleeing felon; hot pursuit
Focal and local
Focal tissue damage
Fragmentation ammunition
Gun availability
Gunpowder residue
Handgun history: stolen, sold, found, traded, discarded, passed on, borrowed, lost, pawned, hidden, thrown away, destroyed, melted down, licensed, photographed, tested ballistically, put on eBay, manufactured, rebuilt, rebored, cleaned, stored
Handgun policy

Hot lead
Irreversible chemical reaction
Needless loss of life
Perforation (what bullets do to tissues!)
Perforation as a verb and a noun
Primer chemistry
Ricochet
Secondary shockwave damage without perforation
Shored wound
Tissue disruption and tearing

Bibliography

Book

DiMaio, V. *Gunshot Wounds: Practical Aspects of Firearms, Ballistics, and Forensic Techniques.* 2nd ed. Boca Raton, FL: CRC Press, 1999.

Research Resources

CRC Press, www.crcpress.com. The CRC annual catalog of publications is a good checklist in forensics for forensic pathologists. CRC also runs a subscription library service to outstanding forensic magazines, periodicals, and journals on an Internet download basis.

Ovid. A private subscription service bought by many medical libraries to establish an easy literature search method. It is available on an individual subscription basis and provides writers with a magnificent service. Your local medical library may provide you download services through their computers. I have used Ovid with a split-screen computer technique and have written quizzes on the current literature with ease.

Note: Don't forget to buy a gun magazine and page through it. You will learn that the gun and ammo data change all of the time. Guns and ammo are just as stylish as women's fashions.

Incised and Stab Wounds

15

Objectives

1. Describe the theoretical pathophysiological changes seen in stab wounds. Describe air embolism and hemorrhagic loss, in particular. M
2. Discuss the following reparative processes: M
   Repair of a partially severed spinal cord
   Repair of a partially severed nerve
   Repair of a lacerated lung
   Repair of a lacerated aorta
   Repair of a lacerated heart ventricle
   Repair of a lacerated liver
   Repair of a lacerated spleen
   Repair of lacerated small intestine
   Repair of lacerated large intestine
   Repair of a lacerated bladder
3. Discuss mutilating injuries of the genitalia: self-inflicted, sadistic, and traumatic. M
4. Discuss the meaning of the term *patterned incised wounds*. M
5. Discuss the incised wounds seen in manic homicides. Distinguish organized and disorganized patterns. M
6. Discuss the methods for the estimation of hemorrhagic loss. M
7. Discuss the methods for the determination of a postpartum hemoglobin and hematocrit. M
8. Discuss the meaning of the words *primary intentional repair* and *secondary intentional repair.*
9. Compare and contrast wounds from the following instruments: cleavers, axes, saws, hatchets, hunting knives, kitchen knives, razors, icepicks, carpenters tools, plumbers tools, burglars tools.
10. Discuss the sequence of events with the death from a penetrating glass windowpane. What is safety glass? M
11. Discuss the pattern seen on bodies with glass injuries. M
12. What are Langer's lines and what meaning do they have in forensic pathology? M
13. Discuss the evidentiary techniques available to the pathologist at the autopsy of patients dying with stab wounds. M

14. Discuss the elasticity component of the human body and tissues. Relate tissue elasticity to the length and depth of a stab wound inflicted in a homicide. M

15. Discuss the phenomenon of immediate and delayed laceration and incision of the epithelial, muscular, and connective tissues of the body. M

16. Distinguish between a laceration and an incised wound. How can you tell the difference between an accurately placed wound and a precisionally placed wound? M

17. Discuss the morbidity and mortality from hemopneumothorax, hemothorax, and hemopericardium. M

18. Discuss the management techniques for single stab wounds of the abdominal cavity. M

19. Discuss what is meant by the term *defense wounds*. Where are they usually situated and what is their character?

20. Discuss the incised wounds caused by razor sharp objects used in suicide and homicide cases, and indicate their relative occurrence. M

21 Indicate the pathophysiology of exsanguination as a mechanism of death. M

22. Discuss the usual pattern of tissue damage seen in suicidal self-inflicted suicidal incised wounds of the neck and of the extremities.

23. Describe the usual changes seen in automobile windshield accidents. Contrast these with mutilating homicidal wounds.

24. Indicate the mechanism of death in air embolism cases and indicate some methods of distinction of this form of death. M

25. Indicate the usual pattern of stab wounds seen in a knife-wielding assailant with an unarmed victim. M

26. Describe the mechanism of death in stab wounds from "exotic weapons" such as darts or spears. M

27. Discuss the postmortem mutilation of the body with sharp instruments. M

28. Describe the terminal actions of an adult dying from internal and external blood loss. Differentiate when there is either slow or fast loss of blood. M

29. How is blood loss treated in the hospital emergency room? At the scene of the stabbing/cutting? What are the various methods of estimating the actual blood loss? M

30. If the broken-off blade of a knife is found in a body, who retains possession? The autopsy surgeon, the coroner or medical examiner, the homicide detective, the homicide bureau, or the police property room? Does the finding appear in the autopsy protocol? Does the autopsy protocol include the broken blade if it is found outside of the body? Are pictures of the blade included with the autopsy protocol? M

Vocabulary

Acute hemorrhagic shock
Air embolism and sudden collapse
Fifteen-gauge needle with IV tubing and saline
Intratibial blood transfusion
Regional blood bank
Sudden collapse due to blood loss
Sudden collapse due to gram-negative sepsis
Venous cutdown

Bibliography

Anderson, W. R. *Forensic Sciences in Clinical Medicine: A Case Study Approach.* Philadelphia: Lippincott-Raven, 1998.

Lew, E., and Matshes, E. Sharp force injuries. In *Forensic Pathology: Principles and Practice,* edited by D. Dolinak, E. Matshes, and E. Lew, Chapter 6. Burlington, MA: Elsevier, 2005.

Spitz, W. U., and Spitz, D. J., eds. *Spitz and Fisher's Medicolegal Investigation of Death: Guidelines for the Application of Pathology to Crime Investigation.* 4th ed. Springfield, IL: C.C. Thomas, 2006.

Whitwell, H. L., ed. *Forensic Neuropathology.* New York: Oxford University Press, 2005.

Asphyxiation

16

Objectives

1. Compare and contrast asphyxia with anoxia. M
2. Describe the four stages of asphyxia: dyspnea, convulsions, apnea, and final complete respiratory paralysis. M
3. Describe the lesions found at autopsy in a case of asphyxia. M
4. Compare and contrast a case of asphyxia with a case on inverted postmortem stasis of blood. M
5. Describe the methods for distinguishing upper airway passage obstruction. Indicate the mechanisms of asphyxiation in the following circumstances: M
   Death in a sand pile
   Bodies found in urban bomb debris (London 1940s)
   Natural gas asphyxiation (domestic)
   Smothering
   Suffocation
   Strangulation
   Drowning
6. Compare and contrast the various forms of strangulation including hanging, strangulation by ligature, and manual strangulation. M
7. Indicate the rate of patterned abrasions and their distinction in cervical injuries. M
8. Define suffocation and contrast smothering with choking. M
9. Indicate the pathophysiology of the so-called café coronary. M
10. Discuss the sequel of compression injuries to the chest wherein it is impossible for the victim to expand the chest for respiration (mechanical asphyxia, positional asphyxia). M
11. Compare and contrast fresh water and salt water drowning. M
12. Compare and contrast drowning with wet lungs and with dry lungs. M
13. Discuss the various tests available for the detection of drowning utilizing blood and other body fluids. M
14. Discuss the phenomenon of animal feeding and drowning cases. M
15. Discuss the body position changes in the usual fresh water drowning. M

16. Define throttling. Indicate the autopsy findings in a case of throttling. M
17. Discuss the mechanism of fracture of the laryngeal cartilages. M
18. Demonstrate the skill of laryngeal dissection. S
19. Discuss the nature of choking incidents and relate them to the passage of stomach contents to the upper airways during the transport of the body. M
20. Discuss the methods by which immersed decomposed bodies can be studied in the instance of drowning. M
21. Indicate the theoretical reason for considering carbon dioxide, carbon monoxide, hydrogen sulfide, nitrogen, and other gases as asphyxiating gases. M
22. Discuss the classification of sternutators and indicate their toxicological and pathological changes.
23. What is meant by the term *vesicant*? What is meant by the term *lacrimator*? M
24. Give an instance of death from carbon dioxide and indicate the relative speed of collapse upon exposure. M
25. Give a typical history for a domestic carbon monoxide death. Indicate whether the death may be rapid or slow. Give a rough estimation of how many parts of carbon monoxide per million in the air will cause symptoms. M
26. Describe the gross pathological findings in cases of slight, moderate, and maximal carbon monoxide retention. M
27. Discuss the findings in the brain in carbon monoxide poisoning. M
28. Indicate the usual circumstances in these carbon monoxide deaths, for example, suicidal, homicidal, and undetermined.
29. Discuss the toxicological nature of hydrogen sulfide and indicate where it might be found in forensic practice. M
30. Indicate the nature of nitrous oxide as an acute or delayed poison. M
31. Discuss the relationship of lung irritants to the development of acute pneumonia and delayed respiratory death. M
32. When a person is suffocated with a pillow, what trace evidence may be found on the pillow casing? Describe the forensic techniques related to the preservation of this material. What is Locard's principle? M

Vocabulary

Blister agent
Café coronary
Fractured teeth

Inner mouth lacerations
Lacrimator
Lip lacerations
Muffled sounds
Petechia
Sternutator
Tongue bite marks
Vesicant (blister gas)

Bibliography

Adelson, L. *The Pathology of Homicide*. Springfield, IL: C.C. Thomas, 1974.

Camps, F. E. *Gradwhol's Legal Medicine*. 2nd ed. Bristol, UK: John Wright & Sons, 1968.

DiMaio, V. J., and Dana, S. E. *Forensic Pathology*. 2nd ed. Boca Raton, FL: CRC Press, 2007.

Polson, C. J. *The Essentials of Forensic Medicine*. 2nd ed. Springfield, IL: C.C. Thomas, 1965.

Spitz, W. U., and Spitz, D. J., eds. *Spitz and Fisher's Medicolegal Investigation of Death: Guidelines for the Application of Pathology to Crime Investigation*. 4th ed. Springfield, IL: C.C. Thomas, 2006.

Blunt Force Injuries and Pediatric Homicide 17

Objectives

1. Discuss and describe the morphology of blunt force injuries as caused by: M
   Jarring of bodies and tissues
   Crushing of bodies and tissues
   Tearing of bodies and tissues
2. Explain the mechanism of death in those blunt force injuries that cause fat emboli. M
3. Indicate what neurological defects are commonly associated with fat emboli. M
4. Demonstrate the skill of frozen section, especially on fat emboli. S
5. Describe the healing stages of a subcutaneous contusion. Define a *patterned contusion*. M
6. Distinguish between a patterned abrasion and a patterned laceration. M
7. Identify various objects that can leave patterned abrasions, include burglar tools such as flashlights, screw drivers, hand saws, glass cutters, pry bars, jack handles, chisels, ropes, cables, leather belts, electric wire cutters, and spotlights. M
8. Compare the antemortem and the postmortem contusion. Discuss the timing of death and injuries in infants and young children. M
9. Describe what is meant by an annular avulsion of the skin of the leg. Indicate the circumstances under which it might originate. M
10. Describe the injuries seen in a pedestrian crushed by an automobile. Indicate the methodology of distinguishing between pedestrians who were hit by a car while in an upright posture and those who were prone on the highway and run over. M
11. Discuss the most modern interpretations and explanations (pathophysiological) for the following complications of blunt trauma: M
    Shock
    Hemorrhage
    Infection
    Thrombosis
    Embolism

12. Discuss the boney injuries seen in a suicidal jumper landing on hard pavement from an eight-story height. M
13. Compare these injuries to someone who was unconscious prior to their fall from the height. M
14. Discuss the elastic rebound properties of the human body. M
15. Indicate a source for elasticity measurements of the various tissues of the human body. M
16. Indicate the "fixed points" of the abdominal cavity and where traumatic mucosal tears will occur in relationship to the fixed points. M
17. Indicate the effects of compression of the chest as seen in automobile traffic injuries. Point to the specific anatomical areas that would tear under such compressive blunt force. M
18. Discuss compressive injuries of the heart (nonpenetrating and blunt). Distinguish the various areas of the heart's anatomy that can be affected by such trauma. M
19. Discuss the complications of closed chest trauma. M
20. Explain the various mechanisms causing traumatic subcutaneous emphysema. M
21. Outline the pathophysiological steps in the development of diffuse emphysema from a tracheostomy site. M
22. Enumerate the blunt trauma changes that may be discovered in the posterior mediastinum. M
23. Discuss the mechanisms of closed head injury and the immediate subacute and chronic changes arising from repetitive subconcussive trauma. M
24. Delineate the various patterns of injuries seen in blunt trauma to the following organs: liver, spleen, kidney, adrenals, and bladder. M
25. What is the major traumatic lesion of the prostate and how is it controlled? M
26. Distinguish Mallory–Weiss syndrome from Boerhaave's syndrome. M
27. Present a classification of the fractures of the skull. Indicate their frequency and severity. M
28. Describe the various mechanisms of cerebral edema. Indicate the relationship of blunt trauma to the phenomenon of cerebral swelling. M
29. What is the acknowledged mechanism for cerebral swelling? M
30. Discuss the timing of the epidural and subdural hemorrhages and indicate their diagnostic meaning. M
31. Compare and contrast a traumatic subarachnoid hemorrhage from a naturally occurring one. Interrelate with this the phenomena of traumatic rupture of a cerebral aneurysm. M
32. Indicate the pathophysiological changes seen in whiplash injuries of the upper spine. M
33. Demonstrate an appropriate maneuver to present the proper evidence for cervical subluxation. S

34. What are the appropriate dissection methods for the autopsy of an anterior cervical spinal injury? S
35. Discuss the phenomenon of spinal cord injury without spinal fracture. M
36. Compare the changes seen with tuberculosis of the spine, neoplasms of the spine, and traumatic injuries of the spine. M
37. Discuss the evidentiary value in the analysis of child abuse of the following: bite marks, swollen skeletal injuries, burns, alopecia, scalp hemorrhages, scalp contusions, orofacial trauma, evidence of starvation or malnutrition.

Vocabulary

Abdominal trauma
Asphyxiation, mechanical and compression
Blunt force injuries: hitting, kicking, dropping, swinging
Causes of death
Choking
Death timing
Drowning
Forensic diagnosis: identity, physiological, pathological
Head injury: closed and open, intentional and accidental
Injury and wound timing
Poisoning and genetic disease
Poisoning problems
Starvation and dehydration
Suffocation, intentional and accidental

Bibliography

Anderson, W. R. *Forensic Sciences in Clinical Medicine: A Case Study Approach.* Philadelphia: Lippincott-Raven, 1998.
Dolinak, D., Matshes, E., and Lew, E. *Forensic Pathology: Principles and Practice.* Burlington, MA: Elsevier, 2005.
Griest, K. *Pediatric Homicide: Medical Investigation.* Boca Raton, FL: CRC Press, 2009, 232 pp.
Spitz, W. U., and Spitz, D. J., eds. *Spitz and Fisher's Medicolegal Investigation of Death: Guidelines for the Application of Pathology to Crime Investigation.* 4th ed. Springfield, IL: C.C. Thomas, 2006.
Stocker, J. T., Dehner, L. P., and Husain, A. N. *Pediatric Pathology.* Philadelphia: Walters Kluwer, 2011, pp. 1–1298. See Chapter 7, Pediatric Forensic Pathology, by Tracey Corey and Kim Collins, pp. 252–271.

Electrical and Thermal Injury

18

Objectives

1. Define the following: Ohm's law, polarity, semiconductor, induction, volt, magnetic flux, electromagnetic field, electromagnetic force, ampere. M
2. Describe the findings in a typical death from lightning. M
3. Describe the typical histological changes seen with electrical burns and define their specificity. M
4. Describe the difference between a low-tension and a high-tension injury (voltage). M
5. Describe the mechanism of death from the following: lightning, Roentgen rays (x-rays), household appliances. M
6. Give a medical injury classification of burns, histological and for an individual. M
7. Compare and contrast the following: a hot dry air injury versus a hot wet air injury. M
8. Distinguish between heat stroke and heat exhaustion. M
9. Describe the problem of summertime deaths of aged people in large cities. Discuss the importance of proper certification of death in a public health aspect. M
10. Define the utilization of the autopsy in the proper certification of summer heat associated deaths. What specific procedures are available? M
11. Compare and contrast patients dying with the therapeutic effects of radiation with those who have been exposed to accidental massive radiation. M
12. What is meant by the term *malignant hyperthermia* and what is its importance in forensic pathology? M

Vocabulary

Accidental massive radiation
Active oxygen species

Air quality
Climatic change
Fatal head injury
Heat exhaustion
Heat stroke
High-tension injury
Hyperthermia
Ionizing radiation
Radiation burn
Radiation necrosis
Ultraviolet radiation

Bibliography

Rosen, C. F. Ultraviolet radiation. In *Pathology of Environmental and Occupational Disease*, edited by J. E. Craighead, Chapter 10. St. Louis, MO: Mosby, 1995.

Gas Asphyxiation

19

1. Review the pathophysiology of the following conditions: M
   High-altitude apnea
   The bends (decompression sickness)
   High-pressure hypoxia
2. Describe the sequence of events in the utilization of a high-pressure chamber and indicate its medical uses. M
3. Describe the passage of gas at the alveolar membrane and discuss the chloride shift. M
4. Identify and define the following terms: M
   Vital capacity
   Inspiratory reserve volume
   Expiratory reserve volume
   Residual volume
   Total lung capacity
5. Define the following terms used with ventilation: M
   Chemoreceptor
   Diffusion gradient
   Oxygen dissociation curve
6. Distinguish the following terms: M
   Primary hypoxia (anoxic hypoxia)
   Hemic hypoxia (anemic hypoxia)
   Circulatory hypoxia (stagnant hypoxia)
   Histotoxic anoxia
7. Describe the pathophysiology and pathological findings in oxygen toxicity. M
8. Describe the usual course of events in the hospital induction of gaseous anesthesia. M
9. Discuss the pathophysiology of the following conditions: M
   Mountain sickness
   Pulmonary embolism
   Asthma
10. Compare and contrast the pathophysiological effects of carbon monoxide gas and carbon dioxide gas. M
11. Indicate a situation in where there is a natural environmental buildup of carbon dioxide. What is the danger? M

12. Discuss the rapidity of collapse in gaseous poisoning. M

13. Discuss and compare the postmortem findings in those dying from acute asphyxia, carbon monoxide poisoning, and hydrogen sulfide poisoning. M

14. Indicate the various suicidal behavioral patterns that are found when carbon monoxide is used as the toxic agent. M

15. Indicate the history of the development of various methods of identifying and quantitating carbon monoxide poisoning. M

16. Discuss the basic pathophysiology of carbon monoxide poisoning including the work of Leo Goldbaum of the Armed Forces Institute of Pathology. M

17. Give an expression of the percent of hemoglobin in combination with carbon monoxide in relationship to the physiological effect. M

18. Discuss the gases produced in house fires and compare the various components of house fire gas in terms of lethality and physiological effect. M

19. List and compare gases that have no remarkable odor and those that do have a remarkable scent. M

20. Discuss scuba diving accidents and indicate a method for the examination of a scuba death. M

21. Discuss nitrous oxide poisoning and indicate the circumstances under which it may be found. M

22. Discuss the pathophysiological effects of tear gases, and indicate when and how they may be lethal. M

23. Discuss mustard gas (pyrite) and indicate its mode of action and exposure consequences. M

24. Define several known methods for homicide by means of gas poisoning. M

25. Discuss the various sources of domestic carbon monoxide poisoning with the photography of the undisturbed scene. M

26. Discuss the care pattern of delayed deaths that may occur in hospitals when the primary insult to the lungs by a lethal gas is several days prior to admittance and treatment. M

Vocabulary

Acute laryngeal edema
Asphyxia
Central depression by drugs
Disaster management
Gagging with ligature
Iatrogenic dissection artifacts

Interference with gaseous exchange
Laryngeal skeletal anatomy
Neck dissection exposure
Obstructive suffocation (foreign body)
Pneumothorax
Positional asphyxia
Postictal respiratory failure
Pseudostrangulation syndrome
Respiration
Signs of resuscitation
Sudden death
Suffocation
Tight collar artifact

Bibliography

Armstrong, E. J., and Erskine, K. L. *Water-Related Death Investigation: Practical Methods and Forensic Applications*. Boca Raton, FL: CRC Press, 2011.

Byard, R. W., Sauvageau, A., Boghossian, E. Commentary on the classification of asphyxia: The need for standardization. *Journal of Forensic Sciences* 56, no. 1 (2011): 264.

Guyton, A. C., and Hall, J. E. *Guyton and Hall Textbook of Medical Physiology*. 12th ed. Philadelphia: Saunders, 2011.

Houghton, R. *Field Confirmation Testing for Suspicious Substances*. Boca Raton, FL: CRC Press, 2009.

Occupational Diseases 20

The forensic sciences are no different from other groups and neglect occupationally derived defects. The pathological changes secondary to occupational causes are often critical to the understanding of the life and death of a person.

Objectives

1. Identify the following:
   Polymer fume fever
   Occupational acroosteolysis
   Vinyl chloride
   Polyvinyl chloride and liver angiosarcoma
   Cadmium neuropathy and osteomalacia
   Chloromethyl ether lung cancer
   Benzopyrene and 6-methyl benzopyrene
   Minamata disease
   Toxic peripheral neuropathy
   Halo-ether respiratory carcinoma
2. What is meant by the term *threshold limit values*? What is its use in safety management?
3. Identify the pathophysiological mechanisms for the following changes due to pollutants: M
   Loss of hair in arsenic poisoning
   Ferruginous body in asbestos inhalation
   Thyroid disease in barium poisoning
   Brain damage in boron poisoning
   Hypertension, emphysema, and osteoporosis in cadmium poisoning
   Carboxyhemoglobin formation in carbon monoxide poisoning
   Nasal irritation in the instance of chromium poisoning
   Thyroid disease, asthma, and myocardial disease in the instance of cobalt poisoning
   Macular skin changes and dental fluorosis with fluoride poisoning
   Siderosis with iron poisoning

Anemia, gastrointestinal symptoms, and encephalopathy with lead poisoning

Rotten egg odor with hydrogen sulfide

Ataxia and tremor with manganese poisoning

Tremor with mercury poisoning

Nasal irritation with nickel carbonate

Cyanosis after nitrate poisoning

Eye irritation with ozone poisoning

Silicosis with quartz inhalation

Garlic odor with tooth decay in selenium poisoning

Garlic-like odors with tellurium poisoning

Respiratory symptoms with vanadium poisoning

Fever with zinc poisoning

4. Discuss the mechanism of poisoning with agricultural organophosphates. M

5. Indicate a laboratory test that would be applicable to organophosphate detection. M

6. Indicate which government agencies are related to the enforcement of rules of safety regarding work-related diseases. M

7. Give some examples of the application of Huber's Law, which is D.T. = K. M

8. In dealing with occupational deaths, indicate the medical examiner's/coroner's investigatory capacity to search other physician's records or hospital records in these matters. M

9. Make a brief statement of the relationship of the medical investigation team in a medical examiner's office to the local occupational health board. M

10. Indicate the nature of the occupational diseases in the following employment groups:

Gasoline station attendants

Hog farmers

Petroleum field workers

Kentucky vinyl chloride workers

Auto seat plastic fabric workers

Pennsylvania coal miners (hard and soft)

Foundry workers

Machine shop workers, punch press

Lead smelting workers

Brewery workers, beer truck drivers

Taxicab drivers, traffic and holdup, and drug trade

Beauty shop workers

Firemen

Policemen

Autopsy attendants
Silo fillers
Gasoline supervisors
Oil spill workers
Electric power line attendants
Home repairmen contracted and independent
Farmers, subsistence and competitive growers
Hunters by weapon and by target
Miners (open and closed mines)
Transportation (air, water, land, teamsters)

11. Indicate the necessity of an autopsy in the instance of someone who has died at work. Compare and contrast this to the person who dies in an automobile accident immediately after work. M
12. Give several data resources available in the area of work-related deaths. M
13. Discuss several references in the field of work-related toxicology. M
14. Discuss the major oil spills of Alaska, California, Florida, and Louisiana, and detail the forensic autopsies of episodic death in man and animal in these disasters. M
15. Demonstrate the collection of environmental contaminants from a(n): S
    Person
    Bird
    Water fowl
    Edible species of fish
    Oyster

Vocabulary

Blood test
CAT scan
Clinical forensic medicine
Emergency room physician
Environmental hazards
Evidence collection in the emergency room
Evidence collection protocols
Forensic evidence storage
Forensic sex crime nurse investigator
Gang violence
Human and animal bites
Interpersonal violence
Personal injury

Product liability
Product tampering
Sedative
Transportation injuries
Urine test

Bibliography

Catanese, C. *Color Atlas of Forensic Medicine and Pathology.* Boca Raton, FL: CRC Press, 2010.
Craighead, J. E., ed. *Pathology of Environmental and Occupational Disease.* St. Louis, MO: Mosby, 1995.

Sexual Deaths and Serial Deaths

21

Objectives

1. Discuss autoerotic sadomasochism. M
2. Depict the usual features of adolescent sex hangings. Discuss the autopsy findings in such cases. What societal values are often demonstrated in these deaths? M
3. Discuss the various ways in which sadomasochistic deaths may be certified. Indicate the speed in which such deaths occur. M
4. Define the following terms: M
   Sodomy
   Cunnilingus
   Sadism
   Masochism
   Transvestism
   Sexual deviant behavior
   Sexually violent predator (SVP)
   Sex offender registration
   Genital mutilation
5. Give a classification of abnormal sexual behavior for both male and female sexes. M
6. Discuss the phenomenon of intersex as a biological phenomenon and a behavioral style. What are the associated forensic problems? M
7. Delineate the procedures and steps in the standard study of a rape–homicide case. M
8. When are swabs of fluids with acid phosphatase of use in forensic cases? Discuss the evidentiary value of a positive swab.
9. Indicate the proper methods for the study of semen in cases of rape. M
10. Why would one consider homosexuality as a factor in a case of excessive trauma to the male victim of a homicide? M
11. Discuss the utilization of the secretor phenomenon in immunology. Detail the serological study of human semen. M
12. In what circumstance is ultraviolet light fluorescence used? M
13. Discuss the occurrence of instant physiological deaths in cases of sexual assault or sexual activity with cervical strangulation or non-strangulation. M

14. Discuss the means of the serological identification of sperm and identification by DNA methodology. Define positive and negative identification of sperm. M
15. Define the following terms:
    Rape and alleged rape
    Statutory rape
    Fetishism
    Sexual molestation
16. Discuss the meaning of positive and negative precipitin tests against human sperm and blood, acid phosphatase studies of semen, and blood group antigen studies of semen in the study of alleged rape. M
17. Discuss the utility of oral cavity examination in cases of sexual death. M
18. Discuss the classification of suicide and homicide cases when the suicide and homicide are combined together. M
19. Indicate the problems arising from the timing of death in the death of concurrently active sexual partners. M
20. How is the pharmacology of male erectile dysfunction drugs problematic in the analysis of forensic public deaths? How do these drugs affect females (erectile tissues in the breasts)?
21. Discuss the role of the waived rapid HIV test in the providing of HIV testing to the forensic science laboratory.
22. Describe and enumerate the mental concerns of a woman who has been recently raped as distinguished from the woman who has had consensual sex. M
23. Discuss and describe the role of physical force in the crime of rape. What percent of rape victims requires hospitalization? M
24. Describe the use of the colposcope, camera with magnification powers, and anoscope in male and female rape. How is toluidine blue used in rape examination? M
25. Discuss sexually transmitted infections, pregnancy, nongenital physical injury, strangulation, and anogenital trauma in the instance of heterosexual rape. M
26. What are some of the common sequelae to sexual violence? M
27. List the usual laboratory specimens from a sexual assault case and detail the careful handling and storage of this evidence (8 items).

Skills

Collection with microscopic smearing and staining of vaginal pool specimens, scrapings of the cervix, dried or moist mucus from hair,

breast and skin exudates, and debris, oral and mucous membrane
scrapings with the identification of sperm, sperm pieces, cells and cellular debris, microorganisms, and parasitic specimens. Photography
and digital storage is necessary

Review of all specimens receiving microscopic examination at medical
and forensic laboratories with photography and digital storage

Ultrasound vaginal recording

Vocabulary

Anal fissure
Assaulted female findings
Bacterial vaginosis
Bite mark castings
Bull's-eye injury
Coitus, copulation, concubitus
Colposcopy
Consensual intercourse
Ecchymosis
Effective testimony
Evidence: prepare, interview, examine, record
Follow-up examination
Genital and perianal anatomy
Hymenal tag and cleft
Male sexual assault
Median raphe (commissure)
Nabothian cysts
Nonassault injury
Patient self-help
Pornography
Posttraumatic stress disorder
Rape trauma syndrome
Sexual assault
Sexual assault nurse examiner
Sodomy and fellatio
Special techniques
Tanner stages of sex maturity
Tears, ecchymoses, abrasions, redness, swelling (TEARS)
Venereal warts
Victorian mores

Bibliography

Books and Articles

Byard, R., Corey, T., Henderson, C., Payne-James, J., eds. *Encyclopedia of Forensic and Legal Medicine*. 4 vols. Oxford, UK: Elsevier, 2005.

Hickey, E. W. *Serial Murders and Their Victims*. 3rd ed. Belmont, CA: Wadsworth, 2002.

Lazzari, M. A. An example of how rural clinical laboratories can introduce HIV testing cost effectively. *Lab Medicine* 40, no. 10 (2009): 581–585.

Lynch, V. A., and Duval, J. B. *Forensic Nursing Science*. 2nd ed. St. Louis, MO: Mosby/Elsevier, 2011.

Ressler, R. K., Burgess, A. W., and Douglas, J. E. *Sexual Homicide: Patterns and Motives*. New York: The Free Press, 1992.

Ressler, R. K., Burgess, A. W., Douglas, J. E., *and* Schlesinger, L. B., eds. *Serial Offenders: Current Thought and Recent Findings*. Boca Raton, FL: CRC Press, 2000.

Seneski, P. C., Whelan, M., Faugno, D. K., Slaughter, L., and Girardin, B. W. *Color Atlas of Sexual Assault*. St. Louis, MO: Mosby, 1997.

Wilson, C. The rise of sex crime. In *A Criminal History of Mankind*, Part 3, Chapter 1. New York: Putnam, 1984.

Organizations

American Proficiency Institute, www.api-pt.com. Offers laboratory proficiency testing.

Medical guidelines for the lab and pathologists are available from the College of American Pathologists (www.cap.org) and the American Society for Clinical Pathology (www.ascp.org).

Infanticide, Abortion, and Crib Death

22

Significant differences in the forensic analysis of infant death and its punishment occur on a global basis. Discuss the international attitudes toward the slaying of a newborn infant (infanticide) as to the culpability of the mother, the father, other family members, and others martially involved.

Objectives

1. Define the following: criminal abortion, abortifacient, elective abortion, therapeutic abortion, spontaneous abortion. M
2. Indicate the size of the fetus at or about the 28th week of pregnancy. M
3. Distinguish between a therapeutic and criminal abortion. M
4. Indicate the steps of proof necessary to convict an abortionist in the instance of maternal death. M
5. Discuss the bacteriological components of septic abortions and indicate the problems in culturing and identifying these organisms. M
6. Discuss the medical implications of impotence and sterility in sexual crimes. M
7. What is a hymen and how are the different types of hymens classified?
8. Distinguish between satyriasis and nymphomania. M
9. Discuss the usual circumstances of sadistic murders and relate these crimes to the crime of prostitution. M
10. Identify tribadism and indicate the forms of activity under this perversion. M
11. Define algolagnia and indicate the activities under this perversion. M
12. Distinguish between a sadist and a masochist. M
13. Indicate the nature of chorionic villi and the architecture of sensual cells during the various periods of pregnancy. M
14. Describe the hormonal changes in pregnancy and relate how they define the gravid state in the female. M
15. Indicate fatal maternal complications that can arise from mechanical (instrumental) abortions. Identify saline abortion, chemical abortion, and estrogenic/hormonal abortion. M
16. Discuss the phenomenon of hemolytic streptococcal infection of the endometrium. M

17. Discuss the changes seen in a case of Bacillus welchii infection in an obstetric patient.

18. Relate the deaths by thromboembolic phenomenon to the existence of septic abortion in an obstetric patient. M

19. Describe the mechanism of death in fatal air embolism from an induced instrumental abortion. M

20. Describe the mechanism of fatal air embolism during sex play of a pregnant woman. M

21. Describe drowning in infants, bathtub drownings, and how to investigate a domestic drowning death. Discuss the parental negligence aspects of infant and toddler drawings.

22. How can a crib death result in a false accusation of infant homicide to the mother, live-in father, live-in boyfriend, or boyfriend? M

23. How did faulty crib design and manufacture result in false imprisonment of live-in family members? M

24. What is meant by the "morning after pill"? What is the latest addition to drug-associated birth control? What is the latest time period for drug-induced abortion?

25. Drug hormonal abortion carries a danger with what unforeseen physiological mechanism? How is it controlled in the hospital setting?

Vocabulary

Cervicitis and septic inflammation
Congenital malformation
Crib death
Drug manufacture chemical contamination
Hormonal therapy of impending abortion
Hyperthermia
Illicit drug contamination
Inflammation-induced delivery
Marijuana smoke contamination
Overheating
Overlying and infant asphyxia
Pillow and sheet DNA studies
Pillow asphyxia
Pillow surface cell studies
Pillow trace evidence
Positional asphyxia in a crib
Secondary smoke inhalation
Sudden death in infancy
Traumatic induced delivery

Unexpected death
Viral pneumonitis

Bibliography

Griest, K., ed. *Pediatric Homicide: Medical Investigation*. Boca Raton, FL: CRC Press, 2010.
Mitchell, S. A. Intrafamilial homicide and unexplained childhood deaths. In *Forensic Nursing Science*, 2nd ed., V. A. Lynch and J. B. Duval, eds., Chapter 18. St. Louis, MO: Mosby, 2010.

Alcoholism and Deaths from Addiction

23

Objectives

1. Distinguish a primary and a secondary alcoholic drinker. Discuss the Jellinek classification of alcoholism according to the Greek letters alpha, beta, gamma, delta, and epsilon. M
2. Discuss the "disease" concept of alcoholism, and compare and contrast the disease concept with the "bad habit" concept. M
3. Identify the following: M
   Acute alcoholic withdrawal syndrome
   Laennec's cirrhosis
   Alcoholic hepatitis
   Acute alcoholic gastritis
   Hallucinosis
   Visible alcoholism
   Tolerance
   Loss of control
   Initial signs of alcoholism
   Withdrawal syndrome
   Alcoholism as a family disease
   Peripheral neuritis
   Alcoholic amblyopia
   Vascular spiders (angiomata)
   Alcoholic cardiomyopathy
   Alcoholic myopathy
   Morning shakes
   Alcoholic facies
   Rhinophyma
   Bottle gang
   Cerebellar degeneration
   Wernicke–Korsakoff syndrome
   Recovered alcoholic
   Alcoholic in remission
   Alcoholics Anonymous
   Diagnostic levels 1, 2, 3 (American Psychiatric Association)

      Delirium tremens
      Dry heaves
      Alcoholic paranoid state
      Acute alcoholic intoxication
      Episodic excessive drinking
      Nonpsychotic organic brain syndrome with alcohol
      Alcoholic hypoglycemia
      Hypochromic normocytic anemia
      Cerebellar degeneration
      Marchiafava–Bignami disease
      Central pontine myelinolysis

4. Discuss the role of alcoholism in homicide, suicide, and accidental death. M
5. Discuss the role of alcoholism in our decision-making processes. M
6. Discuss the role of alcoholism in aggressive behavior. M
7. Discuss the following terms:
      Poisons as the chemical formula
      Absorption path
      Intermediate metabolism
      Excretion
      Physiological action
      Pharmacological action
      Postmortem determination
8. Discuss the following drugs:
      Alcohol
      Barbiturates
      Carbon monoxide
      Intravenous narcotism
      Cyanide
      Arsenic
      Salicylate
      Meprobamate
      Glutethimide
      Propoxyphene
9. Indicate the steps in the autopsy of the patient with intravenous narcotism. Describe the relationship of the following to intravenous narcotism: M
      Malaria
      Syphilis
      Viral hepatitis
      Staphylococcal infection
      Myoglobin
      Uric acid

Nephrosis

Bacterial endocarditis

Pulmonary thrombosis with cor pulmonale

10. Compare and contrast narcotics addiction with alcoholic addiction and with other drug addiction. M

11. Give a short history of drug trafficking in the United States and indicate the international routes for drug smuggling. M

12. Indicate the usual method of distribution of drug paraphernalia and drugs in a large metropolitan area. Compare and contrast the homicide role in drug trafficking to the homicide role in gambling. M

13. Discuss the role of drug addiction to the establishment and maintenance of methadone clinics. Relate the problems of the methadone clinic in a metropolitan area. M

14. Discuss the role of blood alcohol concentration estimations arising from new software programs that are faster and more accurate than former hand calculations. M

Vocabulary

Arsenic

Blood alcohol concentration (BAC)

Cyanide

Daubert ruling

Drug paraphernalia

Drug trafficking

Methadone clinics

Myoglobin

Narcotics addiction

Peripheral neuropathy

Staphylococcal infection

Uric acid

Bibliography

Hlastala, M. P. Paradigm shift for the alcohol breath test. *Journal of Forensic Sciences* 55, no. 2 (2010): 451–456.

Karch, S. *Drug Abuse Handbook.* 2nd ed. Boca Raton, FL: CRC Press, 2007.

Karch, S. *Karch's Pathology of Drug Abuse.* 4th ed. Boca Raton, FL: CRC Press, 2009.

Kintz, P., ed. *Analytical and Practical Aspects of Drug Testing in Hair.* Boca Raton, FL: CRC Press, 2007.

Swofford, H. J. Alcohol in the 21st century: New standards, new technology. *Forensic Magazine* 6, no. 3 (2009): 23–25.

Analytical Toxicology 24

Who is a toxicologist? A chemist out of work......(joke)....

Objectives

1. Draw a flow pattern for the analysis of a toxicological unknown in a blood specimen. Distinguish differences in postmortem analysis, performance drug screening, and urine drug screening. M
2. Indicate the proper specimens to be collected in an autopsy considered to be a death from a general toxicological unknown. M
3. Give the cost, preventive maintenance setup, the duration of production in time, and the usual working protocol for the following equipment: M
    Serum protein electrophoresis
    Gas chromatography
    Liquid chromatography
    Gas chromatography with mass spectroscopy
    Laser nephelometry
4. Discuss the role of crystallography and crystal studies in the detection of drugs. How are crystals used in toxicology? M
5. Describe the qualifications of a metropolitan, "large system" forensic toxicologist. M
6. Enumerate the certifying boards in toxicology and forensic toxicology. M
7. Distinguish between a pharmacological dose and a lethal dose. M
8. What is meant by the term *threshold limit value*? M
9. Indicate the usual personnel and instrumentation found in a 1980–1990 toxicology laboratory. In a current laboratory? M
10. Indicate the problem of pharmacological purity, and the meaning of the term *lethal dose*. M
11. Indicate the problems in the examination of the stomach contents in regard to the following factors: M
    Time
    Passage

Aspiration
Identification of particles
Corrosive action of the contents
Passage time
Autolytic changes

12. Why is urine considered "toxicologists' gold." M

13. What is the meaning of the axiom "every label can be removed." M

14. Discuss the interpretive problems with botulism poisoning and clostridium poisoning. M

15. What are the toxicological and morphological changes seen in patients dying of diphtheria poisoning? M

16. Name three good textbooks on the subject of toxicology that may be of value to the practicing forensic pathologist for case solutions. What sources on the Internet are available? M

17. Compare and contrast exotoxins and endotoxins. M

18. Discuss the autopsy and certification problems in the following types of forensic toxicological cases:
Intentional infanticide
Pediatric ingestion
Carbon monoxide poisoning in a lovers' lane situation
Suicidal carbon monoxide auto/garage situation
Booze and barbiturates in a hotel room
Excited delirium syndrome
Multiple overdose victim
Geriatric rat poison ingestion
Booze and barbiturates in a suicidal psychiatrist

19. Give the major or critical features of the following types of poisonings to include absorption, mode of action, identification, and quantification:
Corrosive acid
Oxalic acid
Chlorine gas
Fluorine
Ammonium hydroxide
Potassium hydroxide
Phenolic acid
Lysol
Metallic salts
Boric acid
Arsenic
Bismuth
Antimony
Mercury

Lead
Lithium
Valium
Nickel
Phosphorus
Selenium
Methyl alcohol
Methyl ethyl
Paraldehyde
Methyl chloride
Cyclopropane anesthesia
Chloral hydrate
Carbon tetrachloride
Carbon bisulfide
Hydrocyanic acid
Benzene
Naphthalene
Camphor
Salicylates
Cadmium
Methamphetamine
MDMA (ecstasy)
Nicotine

20. Classify by giving examples of nonvolatile, nonalkaloidal, and organic poisons. M

21. Distinguish the various alkaloidal poisonings such as: M
Strychnine
Nicotine
Coniine (hemlock)
Opium
Morphine
Atropine
Cocaine
Ergot
Caffeine

22. Compare and contrast food poisonings due to staphylococcal exotoxins, endotoxins, poison mushrooms, food hypersensitivity. M

23. Discuss the cause of death and the mechanism of death in the following bite cases: M
Multiple bee stings
Single wasp sting
Jellyfish sting
Brown recluse spider bite

24. Describe the immunopathological procedures available to the forensic toxicologist and indicate their special specificity. Note the biological errors inherent in the antigen–antibody complex specificity. M
25. Give a demonstration of direct and indirect antigen–antibody reaction used in the practice of forensic toxicology. M
26. When you have a problem in forensic toxicology, which should you do first: consult a forensic toxicologist of your desire or look it up in Wikipedia and tox texts? Explain your answer. M
27. Discuss the effects of automation and tandem mass spectroscopy on laboratory chain-of-custody and throughput. M

Vocabulary

Adolph's meat tenderizer
Adverse drug–drug interactions
Alcohol elimination rate variability
Analytical techniques
Anaphylactic shock
Antemortem course and users knowledge
Antiseptics and medicines with instruction sheets
Automatism
Availability and familiarity of the substance with use guidelines
Bar coding and labels
Biocidal poisons for cleaning and disinfection
Biosafety standards
Board certified forensic toxicologist
Briscoe v. Virginia
Caffeine intoxication
Capillary electrophoresis with laser fluorescence
Chemical assassination
Chemical effect and physical effects of drugs (reactions)
Chemometric techniques
Clozapine geriatric lethal tachycardia
Confrontation clause
Data evaluation, data sorting, data storage
Detection limits
Dissociative anesthetic agent (ketamine)
Drug-facilitated sexual assault (DFSA)
Drugs of abuse
Ecstasy (MDMA)
Electromagnetic spectrum
Fat tissue pesticide levels

Therapeutic drug versus nontherapeutic drug index
Toxicity
Tranquilizer
Urinary metabolite of cyanide, ATCA
Urine adulterant (Papain)
Verifying test and interpretation
Vomitus retrieval
Wisdom of the Internet
Workplace chemical exposure

Definition of a Poison

Chemical effect and physical effects of drugs (reactions)
Lethal dose of poison and victim distribution: data
Therapeutic drug versus non-therapeutic drug index
Frequency of poisoning with official records
Availability and familiarity of the substance with use guidelines
Antiseptics and medicines with instruction sheets
Biocidal poisons for cleaning and disinfection
Antemortem course and users knowledge
Industrial chemicals with catalogs
Target organ histopathology and microscopy
Lesions of poisoning with experimental duplications
Portal lesions, non-portal lesions, systemic changes, and both local and
    systemic changes
Steps in toxicological and chemical analysis: sample choice, quanti-
    tation, sample characteristics, artifacts, instrumentation samples,
    instrument submission, data with automated evaluation, limitations
    and minimal concentrations, significant concentrations, synergistic
    effects, analgesic effect, rapidity of death, intent of actions, motive
    for actions, scene reconstruction
Automatism

Bibliography

Books and Articles

Ballantyne, B., Marrs, T. C., and Syversen, T. *General and Applied Toxicology*. 3rd ed.,
    6 vols. San Francisco, CA: Wiley, 2009.
Baselt, R. C. *Disposition of Toxic Drugs and Chemicals in Man*. 8th ed. Foster City, CA:
    Biomedical Publications, 2008.
Baselt, R. C. *Drug Effects on Psychomotor Performance*. Foster City, CA: Biomedical
    Publications, 2001.

Burks, R. M., Pacquette, S. E., Guericke, M. A., Wilson, M. V., Symonsbergen, D. J., Lucas, K. A., and Holmes, A. E. DETECHIP®: A sensor for drugs of abuse. *Journal of Forensic Sciences* 55, no. 3 (2010): 723–727.

Grey, M., and Spaeth, K. *The Bioterrorism Source Book*. New York: McGraw Hill, 2006.

Hutchkinson, M. *The Poisoners Handbook*. El Dorado, AR: Desert Publications, 2000.

Karch, S. B. *Karch's Pathology of Drug Abuse*. 4th ed. Boca Raton, FL: CRC Press, 2009.

Priesler, S. *Silent Death*. 2nd ed. Green Bay, WI: Festerling Publications, 1997.

Organizations

American Board of Forensic Toxicology, www.abft.org

Society of Toxicology, www.toxicology.org

Labs, Research Programs, and Toxicologists

ATR Spectral Libraries by the cooperation of SensiIR technologies, Aldrich, and ST Japan include a forensic section number 000-0055 with 1465 spectra in a collection of 24 spectra. See www.sensir.com. Also shows infrared microscopy technology.

Alphonse Poklis, PhD, toxicologist, Medical College of Virginia, Box 98-165, VCU/MCVH Station, Richmond, VA 23298

Cedar Crest College, Forensic Science Program, 100 College Drive, Allentown, PA 18104

Charles L. Winek, PhD, PC Lab, 1320 5th Avenue, Pittsburgh, PA 15219

Christopher W. Long, PhD, toxicologist, St. Louis University School of Medicine, 1401 South Grand, St. Louis, MO 63104 (He was my toxicologist when I served Baton Rouge Louisiana. His services were excellent; that is, accurate, precise, authoritative.)

FBI Laboratory, 2501 Investigation Parkway, Quantico, VA 22135

John Jay College, 445 West 59th Street, New York, NY 10019

Michael F. Rieders, PhD, National Medical NMS Labs, Forensic Mentors Institute, 3701 Welsh Road, Willow Grove, PA 19090

NMS Labs, 3701 Welsh Road, Willow Grove, PA 19090

Classification of Death; Therapeutic Misadventures

25

Objectives

1. Describe the classification of death according to the methods of descriptive pathology, the method of problem-oriented autopsy, and by the pathophysiological mechanism with straight listings. M
2. Discuss the logistical problems involved with the classification of death as follows: M
   - Natural
   - Accidental
   - Suicidal
   - Homicide
   - Therapeutic misadventure
   - Undetermined
   - Pending
3. Describe the procedural problems when there are autopsies without conclusive or inclusive findings, "autopsies blanche." M
4. Describe the role of the pathologist in counseling family members as to the nature and cause of death. Indicate the problems that may arise in the family from the classification of disease and insurance policies. M
5. Give several state laws or statutes for the provision of the cause and mechanism of death. S
6. Demonstrate the utilization of the *Medical Examiners' and Coroners' Handbook on Death Registration and Fetal Death Reporting.* S
7. Discuss the relationship of the medical examiner/coroner to the legal report of the office. M
8. Relate the relationship of the coroner's office/medical examiner's office to the probate court. M
9. Discuss the legal rights of the family of the deceased in the actions of the medical examiner/coroner. M
10. Indicate the rules for the relief from abusive situations that are found in many homicide cases. Discuss the role of the social worker and domestic relations courts in these matters. M

11. Discuss the relationship of the medical examiner's office to the police authority of the state. M

12. Indicate the problem areas in the routine management of the affairs of public death and death certification. M

13. Write a protocol for the model method of handling a therapeutic misadventure. M

14. Describe the relationship of the medical examiner/coroner to the hospital committees working in the care of these deaths. M

15. Discuss the role of the forensic pathologist as an "impartial" examiner. M

16. Discuss the relationship of the medical examiner's/coroner's office to the press and television media in the instance of therapeutic misadventures and other prominent press stories. M

17. What is the danger of preloading a syringe with a vaccine, a drug, or an antibiotic? How is a verification of a syringe content made? Who performs drug verification studies? M

18. What drug was verified in the case of Dr. Carl Coppolino, an anesthesiologist, in the death of his wife by injection (succinylcholine)? How was the drug identified when retrieved from the muscular injection site? What principle concerning the solving of forensic problems is provided in this case? M

19. What are the circumstances in which commonly therapeutic misadventures arise in various medical, dental, and nursing practices? M

20. What is the usual mechanism for sudden death in the dental chair? How can anaphylactic death be avoided? M

21. What are the common therapeutic misadventures arising from the following circumstances? M
    Emergency surgery following a house fire
    Schizophrenic depression with electric shock therapy
    Precipitous newborn delivery with an obese mother
    Amputation of an ischemic leg in a diabetic patient
    Administration of methadone to an alcoholic patient

22. What is excited delirium and how is it treated? Discuss the treatment of acute psychotic episodes. M

23. Discuss the physiological changes in positional or restraint asphyxia. How is this related to death from hog-tying? M

24. Show some of the advertising materials you have collected from manufacturers and distributors of the major toxicological analytic tools. S

25. Discuss the steps and analysis you would perform while performing an autopsy on an infant or child who has died within a day or two after receiving an immunization shot. How would you inform the parents and the associated police agency of your expectations? M

Vocabulary

Acute psychotic episodes
Anesthetic risk
Cardiac arrhythmia and sudden death
Child abuse legislation
Conscious sedation
Forensic nurse death investigator (FNDI)
Forensic nursing
Gas line identification methods
Gas tank identification methods
Immediate intervention
Intranasal fentanyl
Intranasal lorazepam
Invented criminal acts
Malpractice insurance
Management of violence
Measuring pipettes
Methadone maintenance
Operating room explosions
Part-time practice
Patient privacy
Spoliation of records
State board of medicine and nursing
Surgical nursing
Syringe calibration methods
Taser death
Undetermined death

Bibliography

DiMaio, T. G., and DiMaio, V. J. M. Sudden death during restraint: Excited delirium syndrome. In *Forensic Nursing Science*, 2nd ed., V. Lynch and J. B. Duval, eds., Chapter 37. St. Louis, MO: Mosby, 2011.

DiMaio, V. J. M., and DiMaio, D. *Excited Delirium Syndrome*. Boca Raton, FL: CRC Press, 2006.

DiMaio, V. J. M., and DiMaio, D. *Forensic Pathology*. 2nd ed. Boca Raton, FL: CRC Press, 2001.

Maeder, T. *Adverse Reactions*. New York: William Morrow, 1994.

Trace Evidence and Criminalistics; Forensic Science

26

Objectives

1. List the sections of the American Academy of Forensic Sciences and give a brief review of the role of the academy in American forensic science. Who initiated the academy? M
2. Describe the Law Enforcement Administration Act and the National Institute of Justice. M
3. Describe the capabilities and the laboratories of the Federal Bureau of Investigation and how they are used by different law enforcement agencies. M
4. Describe the registry of the Armed Forces Institute of Pathology in the forensic science registry. M
5. Analyze a typical metropolitan police department crime lab. M
6. Indicate the functioning of the crime lab personnel at the scene of a homicide. M
7. Describe and list the usual equipment used by crime scene personnel at a crime scene investigation. M
8. Attend five to ten homicide scenes and make a report. S
9. Attend five to ten homicide trials and make a report. S
10. Discuss the use of the comparison microscope and demonstrate its role in the production of evidence. M, S
11. Discuss what is meant by a ballistics expert and indicate sources of training for such experts. List several important references dealing with firearms. M
12. Indicate the use of the spectroscope in the study of paint chip pieces and particles. M
13. Discuss the utilization of trace evidence in the following circumstances:
    Automobile and fixed object accident
    Auto–auto accident
    Pedestrian–auto hit-and-run accident
    Trace evidence and particle analysis

      Rape and personal attack

      Stabbings and shootings

      Fingerprints and foods

14. Describe the physics of the scanning electron microscope and indicate its role in the identification of metallic elements and objects. M

15. Describe the pathologist's role in bullet pellet marking identification, and indicate the usual and proper manner of examination. M

16. Indicate the methods for storing bullet pellet fragments and particles, and indicate the chain of evidence required in these cases. M

17. Describe the role of the forensic examination of the body by x-ray, scanning x-ray, and ultrasound in the detection of abnormalities. M

18. Describe the method for the proper preservation of the following types of evidence. When is a drying cabinet used? M

      Clothing

      Personal property

      Personal money

      Personal treasures

      Seized vehicle

      Fingernail scrapings

      Crime-associated pets

      Personal writings, recordings, and artworks

19. Describe the role of the sound movie camera in the preservation of the evidentiary details of the homicide scene. M

20. Discuss the role, training, and scientific capacities of the following medicolegal experts: M

      Handwriting expert

      Document examiner

      Forensic toxicologist

      Forensic immunologist

      Forensic serologist

      Criminalist

      Forensic epidemiologist

      Forensic odontologist

      Forensic anthropologist

21. Magnifying spectroscopy has had a limited application since most applications of infrared spectroscopy have emphasized the infrared spectral analysis of small samples and do not meet the needs of microscope users. Microscopists have not taken advantage of this new technology even though molecular spectral analysis of single cells is possible. Discuss the relationships of the inventor-manufacturer and the "killer" application, and how a breakthrough application discovery produces changes in scientific methodology. M

22. How can improved methods for elution and extraction of sperm from sexual assault swab affect crime scene and forensic laboratory turnaround time? Give an example. M
23. Discuss Thomas Gluodenis's division of forensic analysis into three categories: (1) Criminalistics—trace analysis, drugs, fibers, hair, bulk pharmaceuticals, and chemical accelerants; (2) forensic toxicology—controlled substances, ballistics, poisons; and (3) postmortem materials.
24. Agilent instruments deal mainly with controlled substances, trace materials, fire debris, ballistics, and explosives. Can you name what type of instruments these are?
25. Discuss the following statement concerning forensic laboratory instruments: a robust data management platform must support high throughput, and activities in archiving and certification.
26. What is the laboratory conflict in the maintenance of certified laboratory personnel and in the keeping of human resource costs down?
27. Describe the coordination of GC-MS with the tube sampler and the analytical software. M
28. Discuss the utility of the digital SLR, which previews UV/IR images through its CCD. (Reference: www.fujifilmusa.com/S3ProUVR)

Vocabulary

Alternate light source (ALS)
Bertillon system
Caseload backlog
Clarification filters for digital images
CODIS database
Context bias of examiners and investigators
DNA expert systems
Environmental health
Expert system software
Forensic epidemiology
Friction ridges
Galton points in fingerprints
Genetic analysis software (www.softgenetics.com)
Hash algorithm in digital forensics
Interviews and interrogations
Lab personnel certification
Laser technology with fluorescence
Low copy number DNA testing
Multiplex STR analysis

Optically pumped semiconductor (OPS)
Real-time polymerase chain reaction (PCR)
Reference and composite images
Sample carryover in cuvettes
Sample processing
Scanning electron microscopy
STR software tools
Surveillance system
Thermal cycler
Woods lamp
Y-STR analysis

Key words in student research after AAFS News May 2010

National Institute of Justice (NIJ) to approve awards under $7K
Forensic Science Foundation (FSF) to make awards
Forensic Science Education Programs Accreditation Commission
(FEPAC) now required for student eligibility for grant money
American Academy of Forensic Sciences (AAFS)

Bibliography

Books

Hood, R., and Sparks, R. *Key Issues in Criminology*. New York: McGraw-Hill, 1970.
Subjects: hidden crime, delinquents, subcultures, gangs, crime and criminal
classification, sentencing, effective punishment and treatment, offender and
treatment interaction, imprisonment effects.
Houck, M. M. *Identification of Textile Fibers*. Boca Raton, FL: CRC Press, 2009.
Koehler, S. A., and Brown, P. A. *Forensic Epidemiology*. Boca Raton, FL: CRC Press, 2010.
The role of forensic epidemiology in public health and criminal investigations.

Periodicals

Emerging Technologies in Forensic Science, supplement to *Bioscience Technology*,
Advantage Business Media.
Forensic Magazine, www.forensicmag.com

Organizations

Advance for the Administrators of the Laboratory (laboratory-manager.advanceweb.
com; advance@merion.com) and the Mayo Clinic are both responsive sources
for medical laboratory information. See www.ascp.com and www.cap.org.

Other

Academy News: Criminalistics Section News pg. 23: "Both reliability and validity are addressed in the landmark Supreme Court decision that gave us the Daubert Factors (*Daubert v Merrell Dow Pharmaceuticals*, 509 U.S. 579). Each of the factors points to reliability and validity in a sense; two stand out in particular:

1. Whether the theory or technique has been tested (reliable)
2. Whether the theory has been subjected to peer review and publication (validity)

The Court gave its "opinion" on the need for reliability and validity, and the *legal community* responded by amending the Federal Rules of Evidence 702 in 2000 to include the major points to be made by the Court. Ken Williams MS JD, criminalistics chair.

Recent Advances in Medical Ethics Affecting Forensic Medicine and Pathology

27

Objectives

1. How is the coroner's/medical examiner's office involved in the procurement of tissues for transplantation? M
2. Discuss the 2003 transplant error at Duke University Hospital with a several million dollar judgement and related issues regarding organ procurement. M
3. What was the involvement of the Israeli government with the procurement of tissues for transplantation from the bodies of Palestinian citizens? M
4. Discuss the world market in organs for donation and transplant. What countries are deeply involved in the selling of organs, especially kidneys for transplant? M
5. How much revenue is turned over with a complete tissue donation in an American hospital? How could this figure reach a million dollars in actual billings? M
6. Specifically detail the different organs and tissues now identified as items capable of recovery and transplantation. M
7. Discuss the issues involved in the utilization of crib death babies in the tissue donation activity. M
8. What is the cost of taking a body to a hospital emergency room to have the death declared in comparison to a coroner's/state patrolman's "at the scene" decision? M
9. How does the need for an autopsy to verify a crib death and eliminate other causes of death (i.e., trauma) coincide with the need expressed for tissues vital to the provision of scarce heart valve materials to be used in living infants? Can a compromise in standards become valid? M
10. Is it within current medicolegal standards to dismiss an autopsy so as to provide tissues for infants compromised by the lack of these tissues in vital structures (e.g., the heart)? Is there a satisfactory compromise or workaround in this situation? M

11. Removal of life prolonging equipment (i.e., ventilators) becomes an argument on the issue of medical futility; however, social consensus is limited especially in permanent coma. Discuss this situation and suggest compromises or solutions. M
12. What were the major ethical issues in the following cases: M
    Mary Jo Kopechne (Chappaquiddick)
    1968 Chicago Democratic Convention and the Black Panthers
    Attica Prison massacre
13. Discuss the ethics of programming the time of death in a homicide case where a recorded rectal temperature is used. M

Vocabulary

Advanced directives
Defensive medicine
Deontological ethics
Dying in pain
End-of-life decision making
Ethical codes
Euthanasia and assisted suicide
Health care ethics and reform
Lawsuit abuse
Medical futility
Moral component of decision making
Palliative care at the end of life
Persistent vegetative state (PVS)
Snitching by police as forensic quality control
Technical component of decision making
Tissue donation after cardiac death
Tort reform
Utilitarianism

Bibliography

Bowen, R. T., and Houck, M. M. *Ethics and the Practice of Forensic Science.* Boca Raton, FL: CRC Press, 2010.

Giles, R. C. Improved methods for the elution and extraction of spermatozoa from sexual assault swabs. *Forensic Magazine* 5, no. 2 (2008): 14–29.

Junkerman, C., and Schiedermayer, D. *Practical Ethics for Students, Interns, and Residents: A Short Reference Manual.* Frederick, MD: University Publishing Group, 2008.

International Forensic Medicine and Pathology Practice; Forensic Nursing; Epidemics and Laboratory Identifications

28

Objectives

1. How did international remote Web-based practice begin? What were the chief practice skills present in the initial team? M
2. What is the chief factor in the practice of forensic medicine on an international basis? Discuss the limited number of forensic experts. Describe Interpol and its functioning. M
3. What are the two most common crimes investigated on an international scale? M
4. Are there international limits or license requirements on the practice of international forensic medicine and forensic pathology? M
5. How are the consultant fees arranged in international cases? What makes up a forensic team for a court appearance or international autopsy? M
6. Are local pathology groups and medical examiner/coroner offices involved in international cases?
   25,000 U.S. workers die overseas each year and many have autopsies from local pathologists and coroners both in their land of demise and at a home facility. (No special papers are needed for U.S. citizens save the permission of those in charge of the body.)
7. Are multiple autopsies on the same body really necessary?
   Yes, as the first autopsy may be an inspection of some limited type, the second a more routine organ study autopsy, and the third a more precise molecular level dissection with advanced histochemistry, pathophysiology, and toxicology including neural system receptors (do not consider limited autopsies to be the result of laziness or ineptitude; rather they are more likely the result of valid decisions to conserve time and to avoid unwanted details).

8. Discuss the toxicological requirements for an international autopsy pathology trade.

 Unless one has had complete control of the body and its fluids (meaning complete control over any toxicological specimens that have been taken from the body at any time before or after death), there is always a chance that someone else has a set of tox specimens, precisely preserved, and may refute any incomplete attempt at toxicological analysis. The toxicological studies must be thorough and complete. At today's prices that means at a minimum about $200. And it means a fully equipped and specially manned toxicology laboratory run by a fully qualified and experienced forensic toxicologist. Most American towns are deficient in the equipping and manning of a toxicology lab and provide services which are provisionally limited. *Note:* The same applies for microbiological and viral laboratories.

9. Many U.S. companies work as governmental servants in overseas appointments. Some of these positions are in the forensic sciences. These are private contractors of services that are oftentimes governmental in nature (e.g., public health and safety). Name several of these corporations and give their URLs.

10. What is the name of the gang leader in the different nationalistic gangs (i.e., the Don)?

11. Discuss the 2006 assassination of Russian spy Alexander Litvinenko through the use of polonium-210, a highly active alpha particle emitter and a fatal toxin. What natural diseases are mimics of polonium-210 toxicity?

12. What is the role of the World Health Organization in international forensic science?

13. Describe the methods and limits of paleoimaging.

14. Why is the identification of *E. coli* O157:H7 so important? Can it be coupled with the identification of salmonella, shigella, and campylobacter?

Vocabulary

Chemical criminalistics
DNA profiling
Electronic evidence
Environmental forensic science
Explosive analysis and detection
Fingermarks, bite marks, impressions
Fire debris analysis
Hazardous materials
Individual identification

Ink analysis
Interpol
Questioned documents
Zug Standing Bear, PhD

Key Words

International forensic science community and Interpol
Proficiency testing programs
Public health laboratory performance
American Proficiency Institute

Bibliography

Bader, D. M., and Gabriel, L. S. *Forensic Nursing: A Concise Manual.* Boca Raton, FL: CRC Press, 2010.

Beckett, R. C., and Conlogue, G. J. *Paleoimaging: Field Applications for Cultural Remains and Artifacts.* Boca Raton, FL: CRC Press, 2010. (Question 13)

Daeid, N. N., and Houck, M. M., eds. *Interpol's Forensic Science Review: A Comprehensive Review of Recent Advances in Forensic Science Methods.* Boca Raton, FL: CRC Press, 2010.

Dershowitz, Alan M. Mishandling bin Laden's body [op-ed]. *Wall Street Journal,* May 5, 2011.

Dershowitz, Alan M. *Trials of Zion.* New York: Grand Central Publishing, 2010. Review his explanation of the "mishandling" of bin Laden's body by burial at sea. Relate this body management to the demise of the AFIP in our government/military (2009). Denial of death reigns.

DiCarlo, C. 210 PO and the assassination of Alexander Litvinenko. *Forensic Magazine* 6, no. 1 (2009): 12–18. (Question 11)

Edson, D. C., Glick, T., and Massey, L. D. Identification of *E. coli* O157:H7 in a proficiency testing program: An update on laboratory performance. *Labmedicine* 41, no. 1 (2010): 21–23. Compliance methods review shows increased but still substandard methods of identification.

Lynch, V. A., and Duval, J. B. *Forensic Nursing Science.* 2nd ed. St. Louis, MO: Mosby, 2011. An excellent text.

Pyrek, K. M. *Forensic Science Under Siege: The Challenges of Forensic Laboratories and the Medico-Legal Investigation System.* Burlington, MA: Elsevier, 2007. The author is a journalist. The book should be read by savants.

Urban Warfare and Nationalistic Weaponry

29

Objectives

1. Discuss the role of the Mafia in the history of American crime. Name some other ethnic American criminal groups. M
2. Discuss the history of the development of the Federal Bureau of Investigation and the role of J. Edgar Hoover in developing its predominant position in global police forces. M
3. Discuss the role of Colombia (South America) in the growth of international crime. M
4. What is the position of Afghanistan in the world drug market? Who controls Southeast Asian drug traffic? M
5. Describe the Mexican influence on crime in California. What is the role of immigration on urban crime in California? M
6. Describe the Mexican crime gangs in the Southwest United States. What is their self-identifying system? M
7. Discuss the role of the pimp in the life of a prostitute. M
8. How is the modern urban police department organized to combat urban crime syndicates? What are the principal methods used in controlling drug and counterfeit rings? M
9. Name the principal federal governmental programs in the computerization of crime fighting services. Be specific. M
10. Compare the ballistic characteristics of an AK-47 with a high-powered, long-range deer rifle. Discuss the ammunition, kickback, sighting, loading, and automaticity. M
11. Discuss air safety and functional design in the planning of new toxicology facilities and include air change control, instrumentation rooms, power infrastructure, vacuum pumps, heat management, and energy consumption. M
12. Discuss the recent advances in biometric identification and evaluate their function in international forensic applications. M
13. Discuss the meaning of *racism* in various cultures and subcultures of the United States. Compare and contrast the concept of racism in California, New York, Florida, Georgia, and Texas. M

14. The urban warfare seen in Cairo and Libya during the years 2010 and 2011 transcend the usual definitions of modern warfare. Relate these wars to the management of crime by police forces and discuss the political aspects of urban police work. M

Vocabulary

Bite-mark evidence
Fairy
First responder
Lady of the night
Mick
Pervert
Queer
Raptor
Scene investigation
Transvestite
Tribadism
White cracker
Wop and guinea

Bibliography

Hall, H. V. *Forensic Psychology and Neuropsychology for Criminal and Civil Cases.* Boca Raton, FL: CRC Press, 2008.

Halla-Borrelli, S., and Pettit, M. Change is in the air: Safety and design of toxicology laboratories. *Forensic Magazine* 6, no. 3 (2009): 35–36.

Taupin, J. M., and Vwiklik, C. *Scientific Protocols for Forensic Examination of Clothing.* Boca Raton, FL: CRC Press, 2011.

Waters, R. Biometrics: Eye on the future. *Forensic Magazine* 6, no. 3 (2009): 19–20.

Bombs, Explosives, and Improvised Explosive Devices (IEDs)

30

Objectives

1. What is a booby trap? What weapons are parallel in design? M
2. What is the association between the Appalachian Mountains and illicit bomb production and use? How does this association work in other areas of the world? M
3. What are the applications of explosives in American agriculture? M
4. What are the benefits of the use of explosive devices in urban renewal? What branch of engineering is involved? M
5. Who discovered nitroglycerine and how is he remembered today? M
6. Who discovered gunpowder and what was its early use? M
7. What causes the different colors seen in firework displays? M
8. Describe the routine use of the roadside bomb and explain how it is used in a field deployment. Describe the equipment involved. M
9. What is a "plastic bomb"? Describe the chemical kinetics. M
10. Describe the usual electronic connections of the cell phone or CB radio to the fuse device of a land mine or other IED. M
    AK 47
    hand grenade
    carbine assault rifle
    mortar shell
    tank mounted machine gun M
11. Name and describe the different groups/kinds of fuses for modern explosive devices. M
12. What are the unique properties for underwater explosive devices? M
13. Describe the methods for delaying the time of explosion for a destructive device. M

Vocabulary

Activation by time, victim, and command
Agricultural associated bombings
AK 47

161

Blast injuries
Bomb technician
Carbine assault rifle
Coal-mining-associated bombings
Component identification and finger printing (fuming)
Deflagrate
Detonate
Evidence packaging
Explosion classification
Explosion effects
Explosive device components
Explosive energy as mechanical, chemical, and nuclear
Hand grenade
In-depth examination
Mortar shell
Negative blast phase
Packaging evidence
Positive blast phase
Postblast scene documentation
Scene parameters
Seat of the blast
Tank-mounted machine gun

Bibliography

Graham, M. *Explosions and bombs.* Pathology Session 63rd Annual Meeting of American Academy of Forensic Sciences, Chicago, February 24, 2011.

Laska, P. R. Post blast crime scenes. *Evidence Technology Magazine,* July 2009, pp. 18–23.

Thurman, J. T. *Practical Bomb Scene Investigation.* 2nd ed. Boca Raton, FL: CRC Press, 2011.

Mental Disease, Paranoia, Aggression, and the Central Nervous System

31

Mental health facilities are state-distributed programs and the variation in mental health activities and treatments are on a statewide basis and formula. Most states are using their jail systems to care for psychotic and neurotic prisoners, and most states have a separate small psychiatric hospital that functions as a jail. They are entitled as hospitals for the criminally insane. Consequently, many jail cells contain prisoners who are mentally ill but who receive no close treatment for their psychotic disorder. The status of these criminals in psychiatric treatment is not generally evaluated in the medical literature.

The forensic pathologist is given some insight into these treatment conditions when a prisoner dies following his or her release or following a furlough. Released prisoners are often missed and may be found in the list of undetermined deaths as the circumstances of their functioning are often gray and indistinct.

Objectives

1. What are the common mental diseases found in prisoners? Which are treated with antipsychotic and tranquilizer drugs? M
2. Describe some of the unusual aberrations of behavior found in suicidal prisoners. M
3. How may the autopsy demonstrate the presence of and the proper treatment of prisoner mental disease? M
4. Discuss the occurrence of cerebral edema, raised intracranial pressure, and cerebral edema following trauma in forensic autopsies. M
5. Define and distinguish syringomyelia from hydromyelia. M
6. Discuss the changes seen in postconcussive syndrome deaths. M
7. The functional significance of plaques jaune, old traumatic lesions of the cortex, may be found in the origin of what defects? M
8. Describe the common surgical treatment of the subdural and epidural hematoma. M
9. Discuss the well-known effects (sequelae) of brain trauma. M
10. Relate brain death to global ischemic hypoxia and respirator brain. M

11. Discuss the role of thrombotic occlusions, autosomal arteriopathy, vascular embolism, and cerebral amyloid angiopathy to cerebral infarction. M

12. What is the usual cause of intracerebral intraparenchymal hemorrhage? How is it controlled? M

13. Discuss the history and treatment of a saccular aneurysm. M

14. Slit hemorrhages and lacunar infarcts are characteristic of what distinct nervous system disease? M

15. What sign of central nervous system infection is not a reliable indicator of disease and requires culture and microbiological study? M

16. Discuss the various organisms seen in bacterial meningitis with different age sets of patients. M

17. What organism is present in acute aseptic meningitis? Discuss this. M

18. What are the predisposing conditions for the occurrence of a brain abscess? M

19. Relate the occurrence of chronic bacterial meningoencephalitis to infections with TBC organisms, syphilitic organisms, and neuroborreliosis. M

20. Discuss appropriate methods for developing and maintaining appropriate scientific relationships of forensic scientists with the local public health officials. What quality control mechanism can be used? M

21. A recent death due to rabies was undetected because the treating and diagnosing "professional" failed to connect the rabies with a recognized bite by what common vector of rabies? M

22. What reaction to infection is seen in about ten percent of AIDS victims within two weeks of infection? M

23. How does AIDS present in children? Discuss this and the associated AIDS peripheral neuropathies. M

24. What is the causative organism for progressive multifocal leukoencephalopathy? And the cause of subacute sclerosing panencephalitis? M

25. What are the modern relationships of cryptococcal meningitis in terms of associated diseases, nature of its course and severity, and the changes seen in cerebrospinal fluid. M

26. Prion diseases are a distinct American (Californian) discovery. Discuss the discovery and pathogenesis of this group. M

27. What is demyelination and discuss its various clinical manifestations? M

28. Aggregates of tissue proteins resistant to tissue degradation are commonly seen in what group (class) of central nervous system diseases? M

29. Neuronal storage diseases, leukodystrophies, and mitochondrial encephalomyopathies are united in a common description term as inherited metabolic diseases. How do these diseases challenge

forensic pathologists in their day-to-day activities and how can they present a intellectual trap to the unsuspecting pathologist? Can you cite an example? M

30. How does thiamine deficiency intersect with forensic pathology? By patient type, by behavioral characteristics, and by its characteristic encephalopathy? M

31. What are the common metabolic disturbances that affect the functioning of the brain and central nervous system? M

32. Give a brief description of the effects of nuclear radiation, ethanol, methanol, and carbon monoxide on brain function and the resultant pathology. M

33. Describe a practical solution to the occurrence of occasional brain, meningeal, and metastatic brain tumors in a forensic autopsy service. Discuss the details of the protocol, the use of appropriate electronic patient records, the resolution of the responsibility for the final diagnosis, and the professional responsibilities of the participants. M

Bibliography

Kumar, V., Abbas, A. K., Fausto, N. *Robbins and Cotran Pathologic Basis of Disease.* 7th ed. Philadelphia: Elsevier Saunders, 2005.

The New Electronic Media, Forensic Informatics, Forensic Pathology on the Web, and Digital Forensics

32

Objectives

1. What is meant by forensic informatics? Who has written a book on medical informatics? M
2. Describe the processes police take in examining a confiscated personal computer. M
3. What are the qualifications of a police computer examiner? M
4. What is the immediate effect of pulling the plug or disconnecting a confiscated computer? M
5. Are the guidelines of the Department of Justice on the forensic examination of digital evidence in 2004 still effective and useable? M
6. Discuss data retrieval from the following: M
   USB thumb drive
   SD cards
   Computer hard drives
7. What is meant by an encryption application? How is it used? M
8. How does a triage tool save time in a computer-based criminal examination? What is meant by "live data"? M
9. What is an American Society of Crime Laboratory Directors Laboratory Accreditation Board (ASCLD/LAB) inspector? In what fields are certification given? M
10. What is meant by Boolean logic support? M
11. What is meant by politically correct scene photography?
12. Who is responsible for the security of the scene photographs?
13. What types of logs are kept with autopsy and scene photographs?
14. How are the photographs shared with the prosecutors and defendant attorneys?
15. What security safeguards for photographic evidence are present when a homicide case is appealed?

Vocabulary

Decontamination
Department of Homeland Security
Documentation
Hazardous environment
HAZMAT techniques
Personal protection
Scene documentation
Scene security
Standards for sketches and diagrams
    What is meant by politically correct scene photography?
    Who is responsible for the security of the scene photographs?
    What type of logs are kept with autopsy and scene photographs?
    How are the photographs shared with the prosecutors and defendant attorneys?
    What security safeguards for photographic evidence are present when a homicide case is appealed?
Toxic industrial chemicals (TICs)

Bibliography

Books and Articles

Barbara, J. J., Digital Forensics Consulting LLC; ed. *The Handbook of Digital and Multimedia Forensic Evidence.* Totowa, NJ: Humana Press, 2008. jjb@digforcon.com

Berman, J. J. *Biomedical Informatics.* Boston: Jones and Bartlett, 2007.

Carlson, B. Speeding the digital forensic process: Bringing high performance computing into the field. *Forensic Magazine* 7, no.4 (2010): 21–23. Discusses current data handling technology, evidentiary data access, forensic evidence processing, and password cracking while noting the future with the presence of rapid personal exchange of data through personal devices, i.e., iPhone.

Duncan, C. D. *Advanced Crime Scene Photography.* Boca Raton, FL: CRC Press, 2010. Basic photography concepts with crime scene concepts; photography equipment with scene close-focused guidelines; special topics including fingerprints, scales, impression photography, two- and three-dimensional concepts, night and low light photography, flash with light painting; difficult objects including blood stains, chemiluminescence, laser, ultraviolet, and infrared photography with applications.

Fish, J. T., Stout, R.N., and Wallace, E. *Practical Crime Scene Investigations for Hot Zones.* Boca Raton, FL: CRC Press, 2011.

Lemay, J. *CSI for the First Responder: A Concise Guide.* With CD-ROM. Boca Raton, FL: CRC Press, 2011.

Organizations

ADF Solutions, www.adfsolutions.com. Offers forensic triage tools.

American Academy of Forensic Sciences, Digital & Multimedia Sciences Section, www.aafs.org

Association for Pathology Informatics, www.pathologyinformatics.org

Logicube, www.logicubeforensics.com. Offers hard drive date recovery and high-speed data capture.

TheTrainingCo., www.thetrainingco.com. Offers an annual techno forensics and digital investigations conference.

Periodical

Magazine of the Life Sciences (info@the-scientist.com), with a liberal distribution schedule; 400 Market Street, Suite 330, Philadelphia, PA 19106-2501 (215-351-1660).

The Asylum and the 60s: The Reform of Mental Disease Asylums and the Consequences from the 70s to Today

33

When I first started into the study of forensic pathology and homicide, I had a firm belief that murder was formulated by people suffering from a mental disease best recognized as simple schizophrenia. This simply meant that the psychosis was free of dominant descriptive deviations of behavior, for example, paranoid schizophrenia. Now many murderers do suffer from paranoid schizophrenia and kill those who threaten their existence in one way or another. But many murderers will not show paranoia of distinct character; they should be classified as simple schizophrenia cases.

However, Emanuel Tanay, MD, offered a different explanation for the psychosis of the murderer. My old teacher from Detroit's Wayne State Medical School, Tanay is one of the leaders in the recognition of "dissociation" as being a predominant mental disturbance of those who murder. It is explained in his book *The Murderers*. He classifies murder into specific and nonspecific murder, and into psychotic (crazy) homicide, or as egodystonic or dissociative homicide, egosyntonic homicide, and psychotic (crazy) murder.

To Tanay, egodystonic murder is committed against the wishes of the murderer and is associated with an altered state of consciousness (dissociation) without conscious motivation or awareness. Dissociation (a defense mechanism with altered consciousness in which certain personality mechanisms escape from the control of the individual) is generally not acceptable to its bearer. Tanay states, "I use the term 'dissociative reaction,' which is included in the official nomenclature of the American Psychiatric Association." The term originates with the psychiatrist Pierre Janet who recognized the capability of the personality to have a splitting of some of its attributes or parts. We know it as the split personality.

Tanay sees the egosyntonic homicide to fit with the mental state of the soldier or warrior. There is conscious approval of the homicide. The psychotic homicide is a totally disorganized murder, completely crazy of course, and beyond understanding or approval. His book is highly recommended.

Objectives

1. What does Tanay mean when he states that the act of murder tells of a childhood that inevitably leads to an adult fury that cannot be held back? M
2. Discuss Tanay's argument that children live in a very frightening and threatening world. M
3. Discuss the vulnerability of the child to the changes in the atmosphere that surrounds them. M
4. Discuss Tanay's statement of parental cruelty causing in the mind of the growing child the development of a cruel superego, which prevents the expression of aggression. M
5. What does Tanay mean when he speaks of every murderer being the product of sadistic parent? M
6. What aspects of American military history support the widespread distribution of firearms in this country? M
7. Relate the presence of handguns and the circumstance of homicide. M
8. Explain the dissociative loss of consciousness as a device for the control of aggression. M
9. Why did Pierre Janet (1859–1947) introduce the term *dissociation*? M
10. Explain Tanay's observation that the masochistic husband's act of murder is the result of destructuralization. M
11. Why will a person in a dissociative state of mind not be satisfied by a symbolic surrender? How is the classification of homicide into egosyntonic, egodystonic, and psychotic applied to actual cases? M
12. What is an aggressophobe in Tanay's terminology? Is it a person with an overdeveloped superego? Why are most murderers rigid, moralistic, confused about their own aggressive strivings? What is conscious awareness? Who is unable to express his/her repressed aggression?
13. Why is the defense of insanity essential for the internal coherence of the legal structure? What opens the door for psychiatry in the courtroom? M
14. Discuss the combination of the unscrupulous psychiatrist with the crafty defense attorney as a reality or a postulation. M
15. Relate the "rotten apple" theory of the origins of homicide to the need for gun control. Respond to the dictum, "When guns are outlawed, only outlaws will have guns." M
16. Relate the slogan "Guns don't kill people, people kill people." Relate the presence of firearms to the laws regulating firearms.
17. Relate the gun as a libidinal object to the immunity of the gun from public criticism. M
18. Why do analysts trace the roots of homicide to disturbances in the murderer's childhood? Explain the psychodynamics. M

Vocabulary

Aggression expression
Aggressive overload
Altered state of consciousness
Combat exhaustion
Conscious awareness
Conscious motivation
Consuming inner rage
Ego rupture
Egodystonic
Emotionally destructive (nourishing) experiences
Episodic discontrol
Excessive overprotectiveness
Going to pieces
Insoluble conflicts
Male castration anxiety
Mentally brutal environment
Overcontrolled rigid people
Parental cruelty
Physically brutal environment
Psychic maturation
Psychic torture
Sadomasochistic relationships
Self-anesthesia
Shellshock
Situational psychosis
Societal institutionalized homicide
Strong fantasies of being unloved/rejected
Superego as a cruel and punitive master
Superego disapproval
Symbolic love–hate parent of childhood
Ten-day schizophrenias
Vicissitudes of aggressive drive
Vicissitudes of libidinal drive
Weapon availability

Bibliography

Dolinak, D., and Matshes, E. *Medicolegal Neuropathology*. Boca Raton, FL: CRC Press, 2002.

Maslow, A. H., and Mittelman, B. *Principles of Abnormal Psychology: The Dynamics of Psychic Illness*. Rev. ed. New York: Harper Brothers, 1951.

Polson, C. J. *The Essentials of Forensic Medicine.* 2nd ed. Springfield, IL: C.C. Thomas, 1965.

Tanay, E., and Freeman, L. *The Murderers.* New York: Bobbs-Merrill, 1976.

Epidemics and Public Health; Molecular Pathology

34

The AIDS epidemic had serious consequences to the progress of forensic pathology. No one has written this modern history. The book *And the Band Played On: Politics, People, and the AIDS Epidemic* provides an initial glimpse into the realities enforced by this viral calamity. The damage to forensic pathology by this disease was great and probably is still operative despite the remarkable success in controlling the disease in Western civilization.

Forensic pathology operating in other epidemics is well recorded. The numerous influenza epidemics are well documented in the public health literature. Forensic pathology operating in natural disasters has been properly documented by the many biographical stories left by our courageous medical examiners and coroners.

Northern snow storms
Southern heat waves
Eastern tsunamis
Ring of flame (terror) earthquake

Objectives

1. Describe the formal pathology training of a public health officer. How does it differ from the training of a forensic pathologist? M
2. How does the integration of forensic pathology and public health services take place in most communities and states? M
3. How does the community decide who will run the toxicology services, the microbiological services, and the genetic services for the population served? Should these services be under one governmental management system? Or should it be performed on a business management basis as in some private enterprise situations.
4. Describe the dynamics of the polymerase chain reaction and tell of its expanding use in diagnostic pathology.
5. Direct hybridization techniques are an important tool in molecular pathology. Describe their utility, weaknesses, and strengths.
6. Distinguish Southern and Northern Blot analysis.
7. How would the technology of cytogenetics be used in a forensic laboratory? What cases would be decided with this technology?

8. Fluorescence in situ hybridization (FISH) has recently become more important in medical science. What is the latest utility of this technology and in what field?
9. What is the current major problem facing DNA identity testing? How is science responding to the current issues?

Vocabulary

Acetaminophen
Actinic keratosis
Aerodigestive tract carcinoma
Agent Orange
Aliphatic hydrocarbons
Allergic interstitial nephritis
Benzidine
Blastomycosis
Campylobacter
Chemical carcinogenesis
Crocidolite
Dirofilariasis
Eosinophilic carditis
Folic acid deficiency
Germinal mutations
Herpes simplex keratitis
Interleukin-1
Lindane
Mycobacterium
Niacin deficiency
Parvovirus B19
Polycythemia
Reid index
Silicon oxide
Tremolite
Visceral pleural fibrosis
Warfarin
Zinc oxide

Skills

Disease diagnosis
Laboratory management

Public health assessment
Quality control
Relational database utilization
Software programming
Vector identification
Viral culture

Why Did the Forensic Sciences Become Popular? The Story and Heritage of Ronald Kornblum, MD, Pathologist

35

The legacy of Sherlock Holmes is a great gift to our culture. It was a physician's crime writings (Sir Arthur Conan Doyle) based on analytical patterns used in solving medical problems. Americans grew up reading his adventures and learning deductive reasoning and logic. Next the great works of Agatha Christie and her Hercule Poirot became standard entertainment. The age before television had marvelous adventures with the Ellery Queen mysteries. Television brought us Ben Casey and the first shows of a medical examiner solving crimes. The English with their great theatrical tradition currently lead the world with their serial renditions of police agencies solving crimes through the analytical skills of their Holmesian-like detectives.

But it was Ronald Kornblum who really blew the lid off of the death scene investigation and autopsy analysis of homicidal crimes. I had the pleasure of meeting Dr. Kornblum in 1967 when he was a resident at the Maryland Medical Examiner's Office. Kornblum was an unusual pathologist in that he mastered all of the available pathology disciplines. He had done his anatomical and clinical studies in California and his forensic pathology training in Maryland. He stayed on for his neuropathology boards under the great neuropathologist Richard Lindenberg at the University of Maryland and the medical examiner's office there. Lindenberg was a neuropathologist for the German air force in WWII and had worked on the Luftwaffe crash fatalities. After the war he was smuggled into the United States in an exchange program and immigrated to the United States through Mexico. Dr. Russell Fisher got him to come to Maryland and the neuropathology program of the Maryland office. Lindenberg immediately became the forensic leader in neuropathology. His assistant, Ella Freytag, diligently wrote papers with him. Lindenberg did his large-slice format neuropathology work on a sliding microtome and established an unequalled collection of brain trauma sections. When Fisher went on the road to a forensic meeting to give an afternoon or evening forensic path session he would include in his ten-case presentation at least three cases from Lindenberg (stroke, trauma, and penetrating injuries). Kornblum took this all in and worked intensively with his fellow resident Charles Hirsch, who would go on to lead the New York City Medical Examiner's Office through the turn of the century.

179

Kornblum went back to California and to my surprise took up his practice in the very difficult circumstances of the Los Angeles office. Although the office has a large staff, it has a crushing workload that is never ending in variety or significance. Thomas Noguchi was the chief there and Kornblum worked along with him. Noguchi wrote two books about his personal experiences as a medical examiner (recommended reading). Noguchi ran into the political problems so endemic to the forensic path trade. Kornblum succeeded Noguchi and spent the rest of his career there. His niece Elizabeth Devine studied criminalistics and worked for the Los Angeles County Sheriff's Department. She would first serve as an adviser and later a writer of a great television series focused on forensic pathology and crime scene investigation, *CSI*. *CSI* struck a new dimension in detective stories focusing on the autopsy and the advanced forensic science skills used to solve homicides and identify murderers. (Of course, friends and colleagues of Kornblum can see his influence and experience on the series.) The *CSI* franchise expanded from Las Vegas to Miami and New York, and to also include foreign versions. The show was unique in its veracity and reality to the crimes of the times. Of course, the friends of Devine's uncle know that the influence and experiences of her uncle Ron were the critical element in the success of the series. On the opposite side of the country, Ron's residency partner, Charles Hirsch, as the Medical Examiner of New York City, was managing the forensic pathology of the 9-11 disaster. Charley could not be honored enough for his diligence in carefully managing the problems in that tragedy.

The detective series, in French, was sent to Louisiana from Montreal as part of the Canadian francophil program. This program seeks to advance the use of the French language. *CSI*-like serial programs from France in French with a Parisian background were skillfull and clever, artful, and human.

Detective stories of the Great Depression era were a popular form of adult and adolescent entertainment. The Ellery Queen stories were the most popular and had their own separate magazine. Agatha Christie was a genius and was the most popular writer in the world. The recognition of our English heritage of the civil service was demonstrated by the Sherlock Holmes popularity.

Television visualized the homicide detective and his intuitive wisdom, while the *Ben Casey* series awakened the model of the problem-solving doctor. But the outstanding champion of detective story entertainment was the *CSI* series. The desktop use of the DNA technology and the use of Locard's Principle were portrayed in the placing of evidence in particular places. The series headlined the laboratories and police of four major U.S. cities. It was a winner. Another graduate of the Maryland office had struck pay dirt, this time with the awesome success of a graduate's child in the forensics field. An entire generation of American youths grew up with a deep interest in the forensic sciences thanks to television and *CSI*. Sherlock Holmes took a back seat.

Bibliography

Doyle, A. C. *The Complete Sherlock Holmes*. New York: Doubleday, 1953.
Wagner, E. J. *The Science of Sherlock Holmes*. New York: Doubleday, 2006.

Organizational Complexity in the Forensic Sciences

36

There is great organizational complexity in the forensic sciences; only government agencies have the depth of manpower and resources to achieve a meaningful intrusion into the various sections of the forensic sciences. And even then, government coverage of the forensic sciences is not complete. Ideology and respect are mental constructs difficult to teach and develop. These early years of the development of the forensic sciences were not without significant problems with truth and authenticity.

Forensic science in the Great Depression was a method for physicians to make enough money to keep their practices going. Remember, these were the days before prepaid medical insurance. Only some police and government employees had free care at the city hospital. Railroad workers had free care at the organized railroad hospitals and had their own form of social security. Work for the coroner or medical examiner was an economic assurance plan for many physicians. Doctors were available for the mundane tasks of declaring people dead and informing police of any abnormalities requiring investigation.

This all changed at the time of the Second World War, when the drafting of doctors to care for the 14 million service men and women prompted a shortage of doctors for the public sector. Forensic work for physicians became a minor part of their enterprise while the wages for forensic work remained at levels appropriate for the depression.

The new pathologist was either an entrepreneur with goals of growth and attainment or a skilled diagnostician with goals of conquering a niche in specialty pathology practice. The autopsy and its forensic counterpart began a downhill descent as clinical medicine became more precise.

The opportunities of forensic practice were now career positions in the city and state forensic systems. The Boards began in 1957 and consolidation of technique and purpose began on a national basis. The American Academy of Forensic Sciences gave forensic pathologists a legitimate professional organization.

The new capitalism in personal finances allowed entrepreneurial pathologists to extend their practices beyond their own hospital. Fiefdoms arose. The question of government medicine as in European countries came to the forefront in the late 1940s and a decision to avoid government management of medicine was made. Organized medicine (especially the American Medical Association) provided a strong attitude of disapproval of government medicine. A loophole to care for the disabled and poor was established in the late 1940s as Medicare/Medicaid. Without a popular vote it went from $1 billion dollars a year to $400 billion dollars a year by the turn of the century. America had government medicine, and the work of the medical associations was to make the administration of the federal medical program a tool of insurance companies and not federal bureaucracies.

As the medical societies focused on the management of health care, the medical schools limped along. The schools had no direct medical society financial aid, as the money went into political fundraising. The schools were forced into the research business and fought for the business end of medicine in new drugs, new appliances, and new procedures. The hospitals took over the management of doctor density through residency fulfillment requirements. They managed to maintain an import ratio of about a third of U.S. doctors as foreign medical school graduates despite the fact that only half of the Americans who wanted to become doctors were allowed to do so.

The medical schools were trying to teach the rudiments of the new and highly technical medical and surgical specialties in costly hospitals with enormous expenses. The economic solution lay in the imposition of a debtor status to the American medical student. It was governmental in nature and had been successful at the undergraduate level as well. The effects of medical school debt changed the entire career plan of the graduating physician. Future plans were driven by assurances that the debt could be repaid. Interestingly many foreign graduates had no debt. And Americans who went to foreign schools were eligible for medical school tuition loans in the foreign land. Washington had no leader, either in elected office or in an administrative position, who could speak and act selectively for the good of the entire American medical enterprise. Medicare is without a leader and speaks from the aggregate voice of multiple insurance companies whose profits are among the largest in the country.

Nurses are working as doctors, and business managers are in the place of the physician hospital or clinic director. The responsible doctor is now managed by a business team lacking good decision-making training and capacity. The model of medical service by insurance company is faltering and very expensive.

Where does forensic pathology fit in this circus called "modern American medicine"? The historically low wages of the pathologist are replaced by higher wages, but management by professional business men with production mentalities who abhor problems (the problems being new circumstances that require some thinking and consideration), delays (the delays are time requirements for the proper use and management of advanced equipment and procedures), and inconsistencies (the inconsistencies arise from the variability of time-controlled forensic processes like putrefaction and color transformations).

To scientifically study the forensic phenomenon in a population of dying humans (public death) takes a team of pathologists (five to thirty) as are found in the large offices in forensic pathology. The skills of each autopsy pathologist when applied to a case require appropriate time and conditions. The factual products of the dissection are often useful in their additive qualities and may be lost or discarded when other material properties are not present. For instance, the opening of a skin discoloration may not reveal a significant hemorrhage sufficient to inflict pain, suffering, or significant blood loss. The dissection may reveal findings that have associative utility which is lost if all of the other associated details are not present. We think in patterns of injury. These patterns may take extensive study and dissection to reach a point of conservative correctness and precision.

Vocabulary

Conservative correctness
History of Medicare
Organizational complexity
Organized medicine
Pathology teams
Role of coroners work in 1930s
Role of research in med school finances
State medical examiner
Student loan funds

Forensic Sciences and the Military

37

Forensic practice in the military:

- Major differences: case type, authority, follow up, testimony, case closure
- Major similarities: case type
- The terrorist autopsy: subjective-objective

By the nature of the practice of pathology in the military services, an extensive and sometimes intensive use of the forensic sciences and autopsy is present. The military population is subject to circumstances unique to the military and the forensic techniques can be transferred readily to the civilian population.

Homicide cases are universally present in the human condition. In the military these require precise study as all cases are subject to official service review. The investigation of suicide cases surpasses that of the civilian world and the problem of suicide is a major concern. The military investigation of suicide leaves no stone unturned. The forensic sciences are well utilized.

Sudden natural death is a concern with the physical loading of the young recruits for their first experience oftentimes with advanced physical conditioning. All types of pathological failures are discovered.

The military preoccupation with violence and trauma defines the work of the military pathologist to include all stages and forms of traumatic injury and death. Both military forms and nonmilitary forms of trauma are studied.

Military recognition of the prime function of the science of pathology in problem solutions led to the famous Armed Forces Institute of Pathology (AFIP) in Washington, DC. The AFIP was a service, educational (at all levels of military and medical personnel), and research establishment. It provided the pathology support for all of the military service including the military medical school in Bethesda, Maryland. Col. Frank Townsend, MD, the director of the AFIP (1959–1963), and Russell S. Fisher, MD, the chief medical examiner of the State of Maryland, which borders the District of Columbia, worked together in the 1950s and 1960s to firmly bond the AFIP to the practice of forensic pathology and led to the AFIP becoming one of the leading, if not the leading, forensic educational sites in the world. The forensic teachings of the AFIP and its forensic science support of the autopsy became an international standard. It was my fortune to work with both of these leaders.

Objectives

1. What was the AFIP and what did it do?
2. What were the civilian available services from the AFIP?
3. What variety of homicidal activity is best studied in the military? Why?
4. Why is service as a military pathologist related to forensic pathology training? Explain.
5. Name other federal government agencies whose services are valuable to the forensic scientist and the forensic sciences. Describe their interactions.
6. Name some major sources of forensic pathology expertise available to those needing this service.
7. What is meant by "outsourcing" of forensic matters?
8. What is the role of the individual's congressman or senator in dealing with governmental forensic matters?
9. Describe the routine of death administration when a citizen dies out of the country. What is done if the case is forensic?
10. How do "terrorist" homicides differ from the ordinary domestic homicide? Are there special steps, precautions, and concerns in the autopsy of a tourist? Of a noncitizen?

Digital Forensics and Forensic Informatics; The New Web and Internet

38

Carrie N. Whitcomb, MSFS, of the University of South Florida, led a successful developmental program for formalization of a separate section for digital sciences within the American Academy of Forensic Sciences (AAFS). The multimedia aspect was not the primary driving force for the section, as the problem of assessment on an investigatory level of confiscated computers by law enforcement was the critical problem at that time. Multimedia was added to the section's name since it too was a major source of computer activity.

The development of a new section in the AAFS was a very complicated venture, but the critical nature of the work fashioned its success. The 2010 meeting of the AAFS included 12 pages and 28 separate contributions to the meeting agenda. Papers included the hassles of deciphering the Vista 64 hard drive, new tools for evaluating hard drives, methods for detecting pilferage of hard drive copy, a Digital Forensics Certification Board, methods of power line analysis, photo print response nonuniformity in cameras, management of videographic visibility presentations, new cell phone forensics examinations, cloud computing and electronic discovery, psychological studies of computer crime and criminals, error rates of classification methods for files, and steps in the teaching of digital forensics.

Just as there is big science and little science, big government and little government, there is big scientific computing and small scientific computing. The big computing lies in the large companies providing the services for huge enterprises such as the FBI or the large health care systems (Medicare), or the industrial complexes. Small computing skills are found in the 50 percent or so of scientists who are not members of large associations or who are not employed by the government or industry and work in simple solitary investigator roles. They provide new writings, ideas, and consultations. There were 120 new forensic pathology papers at the 2010 AAFS meeting.

Since the advent of the personal computer in the late 1950s, the functioning of the scientist has changed for the better. I was at Harvard at the same time as Bill Gates. Gates was a lawyer businesswoman's son who was tutored in computers when he was a teenager and arrived at Harvard to stay for only a year because he had derived MS-DOS, the basic language of the personal computer. Gates had to perfect it, make it into a business success, and prove its value to the world. At that time seemingly hundreds of electronics people were devising personal computers, but none could do what Gates did; that is, make a system that could be applied to a simple computer with an operating system understandable to the millions. His contribution was unique and his business acumen after that patent was outstanding. He really introduced computers to the world and dominated the world market. This market had hundreds of electronic engineers but none could hold a candle to Gates. I was thrilled by Gates's discovery and quickly saw what he had done.

Every scientist should have his or her own gallery of software programs that they understand and can use. Microsoft batched together its basic group of software programs into an "office" package. It included a word processing package (Word), a publications package for communications (Publisher), an Excel spreadsheet, a lecture projection program (PowerPoint), and a relational database (Access). Outlook, a scheduling aid, was later added, and those who were into Web design and communications studied HTML and XML with some study of JavaScript. Visio, a program teaching uniform diagramming for businesses and science, followed and was placed into the MS Office group. An additional program was to teach programming on a "basic level" and followed the Basic programming methods to Visual Basic.Net.

Photoshop (or an equivalent) and programs to burn CDs for duplication are part of a scientist's software treasury. All scientists should take on a statistics program, and journal editors often prefer certain programs. At publication time the data is often presented offline on the Web. A personal Web site with recently fashioned reports, evaluations, and opinions is also becoming standard practice for scientists. Recent social networking has added a new dimension and the virtual classroom has now been made a universal. John Minarcik, MD is a particular standout in this new educational dimension.

The point to all of this is that the scientist and in particular the pathologist in the last three decades has had a tremendous burden of sophisticated computer learning based on the needs of the science of pathology, the needs of his own personal scientific endeavors, and needs of the hospital, government, or medical corporation with which he or she is associated. New programs such as Silverlight, InfoPath, Captivate, and Facebook arise almost spontaneously into the realm of the individual computer-oriented pathologist. However, the same aggrandizement of software programs is taking place at the institutional level and institutions are squeezed by the necessities of the government mandates on computerized records and the required use of computerized business practices to operate in modern medical practice (i.e., demands of the insurance companies).

A scientist now has an Internet to communicate through, hundreds of separate computer software programs dedicated to his advancement, a mature and proliferating science informatics network, and a mature personal computing environment to navigate. Both the solo scientist and the corporate scientist using huge associations of computers for the development of ideas and theories are challenged beyond their expectations. The forensic science enterprise in computers has been limited, but the section in the AAFS should stimulate new approaches and ideas.

Objectives

1. What is meant by the digital visual revolution? Explain the transition from film to digital storage. What are its ramifications?
2. What is the relationship of live box analysis to random access memory in forensic computer investigations?
3. What is radiotelemetry and how is it used?
4. What is a wireless local area network and how is it used?
5. Explain the benefits of Bluetooth technology.
6. What technology is used in global positioning systems? Explain.
7. Explain how the governmental drive to establish the electronic medical record (the electronic hospital record) is putting the pressure on medical science to invest heavily into computer resources.
8. Discuss the following statistical packages and tests:
   SPSS statistical package
   SAS software
   Chi-square test for categorical variables
   Fisher's exact test for categorical variables
   Wilcoxon rank series test for continuous variables
9. What does it mean to have significance when the p value is 0.05 or less?
10. How was scene investigation changed by the digital visual revolution?
11. Explain the technology of paleoimaging. How is it used in the forensic sciences?
12. Contrast the relational databases of Oracle and Access.

Vocabulary

Communities of practice
Continuing education
Internet
Social software
Web 2.0
Web site

Bibliography

Berman, J. J. *Biomedical Informatics.* Sudbury, MA: Jones and Bartlett, 2007.

Berman, J. J. *Neoplasms: Principles of Development and Diversity.* Sudbury, MA: Jones and Bartlett, 2009.

Duval, J. B. Digital evidence and forensic investigations. In *Forensic Nursing Science,* edited by V. A. Lynch and J. B. Duval, Chapter 9. St. Louis, MO: Mosby, 2010.

Schreiber, W. E., and Giustini, D. M. Pathology in the era of the Web 2.0. *American Journal of Clinical Pathology* 132 (2009): 824–828.

Organizations

Microsoft, www.microsoft.com

National Institute of Standards and Technology, Statistics Portal, www.nist.gov/statistics-portal.cfm

University of Missouri-St. Louis Computer Education & Training Center, www.cetc.umsl.edu

NIST has a free statistical package that is downloadable, www.nist.gov

Advanced Microscopic Techniques

39

The new level of pathological diagnosis as applied to forensic pathology is designated as forensic molecular pathology. Invitrogen with bioprobes, biomarkers, and special stains are some of the leading techniques in this field. Studies include:

Communication studies
Ion indicators
Calcium-induced cell death
Mitochondrial function and biochemistry
Cell counting and indexing
Automated cell counters
Nucleic acid identification and quantitation

Note: A review of the submissions for the AAFS 2010 meeting in Seattle shows few papers related to the proofs molecular biology can give to the histopathological and cytopathological evidence used in autopsy analysis. In other words, there is a lot of work needed in this field in order to reach the courtroom.

These techniques became of significance to the forensic pathologist when they incorporated spectrophotometry into the electronic beams of their scanning electron microscopes. Elemental identification now became a property of these scanning scopes; it did not hurt that they were much simpler and cheaper than the competitive chemical isolation science and less laborious than the large electron microscopes. The latest papers relate the use of phase plates in biological electron microscopy; phase contrast (defocus and Zernike), Schlieren optics, and Hilbert differential phase contrast techniques are used to find contrast in transparent objects. None of these techniques are exclusively formulated for forensic purposes but are applicable in all of the sciences. The forensic scientist has no limits to his or her discovery skills in pursuing the perpetrators of crime. This is because the criminal acting outside of the law may lead a trail into areas sheltered from discovery to evade detection. We all know the story of the melting icicle as a murder weapon.

Forensic molecular pathology includes these important techniques, which provide important evidence if they are used properly and sufficiently.

Polymerase chain reaction
Direct hybridization methods
Southern and northern blot analysis
Cytogenetics
Fluorescence in situ hybridization
DNA identity testing

The AIDS Epidemic and Its Consequences to Forensic Pathology

The story of the aids epidemic is recounted in the book *And the Band Played On: Politics, People, and the AIDS Epidemic.* A male flight attendant caught the virus in Africa and then deposited it in Europe, Canada, and the United States. A New York City pathologist practicing in parasitic diseases tells the story of how he missed the AIDS epidemic when it hit the homosexual community of dancers in New York. He treated their diarrhea as though it was a parasitic infection of some sort. He recorded their anorexia and stood by hopelessly as they died.

Performing an AIDS autopsy was an experimental procedure. There were no standards save for complete isolation. I discovered that it was difficult for virologists to isolate the virus if the specimen was out of the body for 24 hours. So we held our AIDS autopsy bodies in the cooler for 24 hours. Then I applied the lessons learned at the tuberculosis hospital at The Ohio State University.

I double gowned, double gloved, and double masked. I did the autopsy solo without any assistance, as I did not know how to protect an assistant. The tissues removed at autopsy were put into formalin and the jar sealed. Instead of histology I made slide imprints of the organs and stained them myself. I was able to document the presence of acute infection in the lungs and bronchi while there was exclusion of the infection from the brain and other organs of the body. Using self-performed cytology saved us an entire episode of supersurveillance in the upstairs histology lab.

The AIDS autopsy turned out to be a simple pathological picture of dense bilateral confluent viral pneumonia. Once the pattern of mortal disease was identified in these victims, the autopsy dissection was fast and easy. We did not use knives save for the skin incisions (the torso Y incision and the cephalic interauricular incision); we used scissors and had no contaminating sticks or cuts.

Forensic Molecular Pathology

Forensic molecular pathology is a new pathology service and is not well recognized. With hospital management (and not academic management), the various services are separated from one another; often they have different service chiefs. DNA is separate from immunohistochemistry, which is separate from electron microscopy, which is separate from scanning electron microscopy, and so forth. It is part of our general failure to provide smart people with leadership of more than one diagnostic or service tool. Molecular pathology lab space must be defended from additional space for surgical pathology. The capabilities at polymerase chain reaction (PCR), tissue, immunopathology, and direct hybridization have to be recognized and defended.

Vocabulary

Community relationships
Coordinating forensic laboratories
Demonstrative photographs and drawings
Distractions and evidence contamination
Evidence disbursement sheet
Evidence recovery guidelines
Locard's principle
Victim advocate certification

Bibliography

Books

Dabbs, D. J. *Diagnostic Immunohistochemistry*. New York: Churchill Livingstone, 2002.
Jamieson, A., and Moenssens, A., eds. *Wiley Encyclopedia of Forensic Science*. 5 vols. Hoboken, NJ: Wiley, 2009.
Leonard, D. G. B., ed. *Diagnostic Molecular Pathology*. Philadelphia: W.B. Saunders, 2003.
Rapley, R., and Whitehouse, D. *Molecular Forensics*. Hoboken, NJ: Wiley, 2007.
Shilts, R. *And the Band Played On: Politics, People, and the AIDS Epidemic*. New York: St. Martin's Press, 1987.

Organizations

Advance for Administrators of the Laboratory, http://laboratory-manager.advance-web.com
Invitrogen Corporation, www.invitrogen.com

Microscopy Society of America, www.microscopy.org. Also produces the magazine *Microscopy Today* (www.microscopy-today.com) and the journal *Microscopy and Microanalysis*.

Pittcon Conference & Expo, www.pittcon.org

Forensic Entomology in Forensic Pathology

40

Objectives

1. Describe the biological characteristics of the first organisms to arrive at a discarded dead body. M
2. What is an invertebrate detritivore? M
3. Discuss the interplay of the blowfly and the dead body. M
4. What do dermestid beetles do to a dead body? When do they arrive at the abandoned body? M
5. *Conicera tibialis* is the coffin fly. What is its unique capability? M
6. What is the usual reaction of indigenous fleas, body lice, and head lice when the host organism dies? Explain. M
7. Describe how the life cycle of the fly is used to determine the time of death of a person? Relate the role of temperature in the process. M
8. What are the common methods of insect identification? M
9. What is the fate of human sperm-derived mitochondrial DNA in somatic cells? M
10. Describe the diatom test for drowning victims and discuss its use. M
11. Describe the utility for identification and forensic investigation of a dead person's toothbrush. M
12. Outline a basic protocol for the examination of a forensic wound. M
13. How might eating pastry from a European bakery contaminate a screen for illegal drugs? M
14. What is palynology and how is it used in forensics? M
15. Describe the positive and negative features of the use of rigor mortis in forensic body descriptions. M
16. Discuss the presence and persistence of human sperm—dead and alive—in the female vagina. M
17. Can identification of a person arise from the DNA identification from the fly larvae on the body? Discuss. M
18. Discuss spontaneous human combustion as an entity. What is the wick effect? M

Vocabulary

Climatology in insects
Insect carcasses in preventive medicine
Shortest interval for growth in the timing of death
Species identification by DNA methodology
Species identification by morphology keys
Standardized analysis in scene investigation
Thermoregulation in insects

Bibliography

Byrd, J. H., and Castner, J. L. *Forensic Entomology: The Utility of Arthropods in Legal Investigations*. 2nd ed. Boca Raton, FL: CRC Press, 2010.

Gennard, D. *Forensic Entomology: An Introduction*. Hoboken, NJ: Wiley, 2007.

Smith, K. G. V. *A Manual of Forensic Entomology*. Ithaca, NY: Cornell University Press, 1986.

Storlie, D., and McPhail, J. R. Taphonomy, necrosearch, and mass grave exhumation. In *Forensic Nursing Science*, 2nd ed., by V. A. Lynch and J. B. Duval, chapter 22. St. Louis, MO: Mosby/Elsevier, 2011.

Weedn, V. Postmortem identification of remains. *Clinics in Laboratory Medicine* 18, no. 1 (1998): 115–137.

Clinical Forensic Pathology

41

Bill Anderson, MD, championed the clinical forensic pathology discipline in the 1980s. He started an active service in his Orlando, Florida, hospital and presented several studies demonstrating the effectiveness of the service and the enhanced role of forensic pathologists applying their knowledge to the clinical scene. He promoted the activity at national meetings and his own writings.

At about this time the training period for forensic pathology was extended to two years and part of the pressure responsible for the time expansion was the growing cohesion of patient services with the expansion of the medical specialties and subspecialties. Consultation became a standard practice and the group opinion overcame solitary medical expertise.

The same weakness of the evidentiary chain exists today as in the past. The role of the pathologist in offering precise and exact descriptions leading to definitive diagnoses of victims is a needed and useful one. Each training program should design a system of clinical exposure for its forensic pathology residents that will provide the resident with a full and complete experience. The array of patients and their conditions is large but well known. The objectives will provide an easy index of their identity.

Objectives

1. Describe the clinical appearance of the 9-year-old victim of a house fire who has survived thanks to a last-minute rescue. M
2. What are the salient features of heat exposure and where would you find burnt hairs? M
3. Is smoke in the nostrils of any significance in evaluation of a house fire survivor? Discuss airway smoke particle significance. M
4. Review the rule on nines with fire victims. Discuss the drawing of blood for carbon monoxide measurement and discuss the diagnostic standards for carbon monoxide levels. M
5. Should special attention be paid to the corneas of the eyes in fire victims? Explain. Where are heat changes evident on a living body? M
6. Should photographs be part of the medical record in a fire victim? Explain. M
7. Describe the role of pharyngeal swelling and edema in postfire airway problems. Can the laryngeal tissues also be affected in the fire damage? Explain. M

8. Contrast steam burns with oil burns with burning fabric burns. M
9. Describe the typical skin and bone injuries in a fall of 16 feet from a ladder. M
10. If a hammer is used as a defensive weapon, what injuries may be a consequence of its use? Please describe them. M
11. Show several methods for creating a mathematical map of an injury to the front of the head. S
12. Define a laceration and describe its marginal features. M
13. Distinguish a fall down a flight of stairs from a pushed fall down a flight of stairs. M
14. Describe the stages of discoloration in a black eye. M
15. Can falling furniture cause a laceration? If so, describe its features. M
16. Name the characteristic injuries of belted passengers in an automobile accident when: M
    They are injured by an airbag explosion
    They are seated in the driver's seat
    They are seated in the passenger seat
    They are seated behind the driver
    They are seated behind the passenger seat
17. Cite the dangers of immediate (too hasty) transportation of the motor vehicle accident victim. M
18. What are the forensic responsibilities of the first responder on the scene? Discuss the use of an opening camera shot of the victim and the victim in the scene for medical and forensic purposes. Why would an opening photograph be an asset? Relate to both medical and forensic purposes. M
19. Discuss some of the serious chemical, physical, and biological injuries arising from careless initial entry into a toxic forensic scene. M
20. Compare and contrast the solo individual technique of forensic pathology investigation with that of a team of forensic investigators. M
21. Describe the preferred method and give the usual stages of forensic scene management by law enforcement agencies. M
22. When does the hospital emergency room become the crime scene or equivalent? What is the evidentiary value of emergency room statements and physical findings?
23. What medical and forensic tests are reliable in distinguishing: M
    Pregnancy from nonpregnancy
    Consciousness from unconsciousness
    Drunkenness from social drinking
    Blindness from partial sight
    Dementia from temporary drug effect

24. Describe the common clinical partial or incomplete physical signs of attempted suicide by: M
    Handgun (e.g., revolver)
    Long kitchen knife
    Hanging with a laundry line rope
    Suffocation with a plastic shopping bag
    Aspirin tablet ingestion
25. Discuss the reliability of eyewitnessed events in the matter of legal proof of a homicide, medical malpractice, tampering of foods and drugs, drug abuse, and domestic violence. M
26. How would you collect correlating evidence from the following hospitalized in-bed patients who are victims of violence?
    Swimming pool partial-drowning victim
    Driver of a crashed gasoline truck
    Passenger of a bus–motor vehicle rear-end collision
    Drunken firefighter who fell down the stairs
    Alzheimer's patient who wandered from daughter's home into the backwoods
27. How would you work up and interview a car bomb victim who survived a blast and has survived life-saving surgery? M
28. The famous Dr. Jack Kevorkian, while a pathology resident with me at the Detroit Receiving Hospital, worked the emergency room and did some early work in the recognition of traumatic changes in emergency room patients. His most recognized work was on the retinal (artery and vein) red blood cells before and after death. What changes are seen in the retinal red blood cells after death? How would these changes be documented? S, M

Bibliography

Stark, M. M. *A Physician's Guide to Clinical Forensic Medicine.* Totowa, NJ: Humana Press, 2000. After covering some history and reviewing the principles, the topics are sexual assault, accidents, crowd control agents, restraints, prisoner care, infections, substance abuse, death in custody, and traffic trauma.

Practical Advice for Forensic Pathologists

42

Forensic Pathology Worksite Checklist

Office with communications, library, and storage
Computer with software and printer with paper
Web station with notices and a mail drop
Dissection tools, scales, and measurement tools
Lighting (field and focal), ventilation, and body lifts
Table, sink, spray, sponges, towels, scoops, containers
Specimen containers, labels, numbering system, pencils, markers
Kits: toxicology, serology, rape, sperm slides, stomach contents
Slide kits: conjunctiva, oral, anal, genitalia, skin, powders
Magnifiers and cameras with recorders
Variable diagnostic light sources (UV/IR)
Fuming hood with air exhaust
Soft flooring with spill, splatter, and aerosol protections
Ultrasound and x-ray equipment with recording capacity
Sanitation and decontamination systems with disposal
Trained and certified assistants
Locker room with shower and dressing area
Privacy arrangements with approved security camera system
Closed viewing area with seating
Outsourcing shipping areas with established contacts

Thoughts for Beginners

1. First pass your boards. A job at a university should give you the time to perfect your exam performance. Remember you can work as a staff pathologist by virtue of your anatomical boards and do your forensic work secondarily. If you have debts to pay off, this may be preferred action.
2. Join the specialty organizations and learn from their conventions and workshops. The organizations include the American Academy

of Forensic Sciences (AAFS), National Association of Medical Examiners (NAME), American Society for Clinical Pathology (ASCP), College of American Pathologists (CAP), Association of Clinical Scientists, equivalent British and Canadian societies, and your state and local societies. Work into the leadership of those that you really learn from. It was economically hard for me to justify extended membership in the medical practice organizations (i.e., American Medical Association, state, and local groups) and membership in groups focused on my specialties. Those are decisions of limitation secondary to the overabundance of medical groups. Use these groups for your continuing medical education annual points.

I use the New England Journal of Medicine Continuing Medical Education program because it is very generalized and stays up-to-date. Also I use the applicable programs of NetCE—Continuing Education Online (www.NetCE.com) for the convenience it offers.

3. Get a life membership in your academic heritage: your college and your medical school. If you are a teacher join Group for Research in Pathology Education (GRIPE) and International Association of Medical Science Educators (IAMSE). Experimentalists belong in the experimental pathology groups. Slide readers congregate in the international groups.

4. Become a grant writer and learn the financial needs of your institution or self-corporation. (I do not speak from experience.)

5. Establish an Internet presence with your own Web site. Also follow the news on Yahoo and Google; use their free daily referral service on topics you select. (For my generation, this was a real trip.) Get on your preferred pathologist Web service (e.g., PATHO-L from Ed Uthman, MD, of Houston, Texas). Work on your computer skills and master the systems you use in your practice.

6. Start building your curriculum vitae. Publish your initial pathology studies in some of the respectable journals. Study self-publication. Look into starting your own little journal if you need a forum for your thoughts. Bill Sturner, MD, set a great example with his *Pathology Gazette* in the 1970s when publication was a chore.

The easiest paper for a pathologist to write and yet make a definite contribution to pathology and science is to simply classify the workload of the pathologist into case types and place the caseload into a table. The table can be searched for various relationships (such as the relationship to wealth, taxation, zip code number, sociological dimensions) either by hand and the sorting of the various Excel sheets containing the data. Or the data can be entered into Access and the relationships of the data worked by Access denominators. Of course, the relationships of the data can then be compared with other series written by other pathologists. Not enough of this type of analysis is performed and much pathology is to be learned from these relationships derived from practice parameters. Relationships are derived first from the development of lists and list creation is a craft that is underestimated in its utility.

7. Visit the major toxicology and medical examiner offices in your part of the country.

8. Attend the major forensic and pathology meetings as available.

9. Establish an account at Amazon.com or other textbook retailer and you can secure a lot of great forensic books with secondhand pricing.

10. Look into the pathologist computer groups, such as that of Michael Becich, MD, of the University of Pittsburgh and the Association for Pathology Informatics (API). Check out the American Society for Investigative Pathology (ASIP).

11. No one told me to learn Microsoft Access. I just stumbled upon it as part of Microsoft Office package; but I will tell you that as an analyst you have to have command of statistics and the use of a relational database. The database systems above the Access format (such as Oracle and SQL) require licensing of the users, which is generally too complicated for academic situations. Access is an essential software for the analytical pathologist as it is the cheapest and most readily available relational database. A self-teaching module for Access is present in the Professional edition. Community college programs often teach it at several levels. The program is a step above MS Excel, which everyone commonly knows.

12. You will need a surgical path godfather for your tough cases. You can find someone commercially, use someone from your residency, or use the local guru. You will need help and do not be embarrassed by asking.

13. And in the words of Tommy Igoe of New York, my drumming (percussion) teacher: "Be sure to have fun."

14. The easiest paper for a pathologist to write and yet make a definite contribution to pathology and science is to simply classify the workload of the pathologist into case types and place the case load into a table. The table can be searched for various relationships (such as the relationship to wealth, taxation, zip code number, sociological dimensions) either by hand or the sorting of the various Excel sheets containing the data. Or the data can be entered into Access and the relationships of the data worked by Access denominators. Of course, the relationships of the data can then be compared with other series written by other pathologists. Not enough of this type of analysis is performed and much pathology is to be learned from these relationships derived from practice parameters. Relationships are derived

firstly from the development of lists, and list creation is a craft which is underestimated in its utility.

15. The analysis of practice contents leads readily into forensic epidemiology. Forensic epidemiology is explained by a well written chapter in Lynch's *Forensic Nursing Science* (Chapter 4: Forensic Epidemiology and the Forensic Nurse by Steven A. Koehler, PhD, MPH) and emphasizes that forensic epidemiology started out with the investigation of terrorist activities with the methods of public health system epidemiology. A wider definition of forensic epidemiology arrives with the concept of public death bearing the forensic attributes to the general public problem of death. A wide area of interchange of ideas is present when the concepts of forensic epidemiology are related to human sociology. Sociology is the academic home of criminalistics and its associated fields. In many state scientific academies and in many universities, the sociology department provides guidance to the criminalistics section. Harvard's E.O. Wilson, PhD presented the human aspects of social biology in the last chapter of his book *Sociobiology, The New Synthesis* several decades ago. He translated his biological experiences with colonial ants to the culture and learning behavior of human beings. Insights from this kind of experience and type of study provide important clues to the basic attributes of the common sociology of murder. Emanuel Tanay provides this type of analysis in his book *The Murderers* (see Chapter 33).

Before You Start an Autopsy: Things to Do and Think About

Clear legal basis with agreed course of action in procedures
Clean ethics
Original patient records including dental records (at least on order)
Identification with forensic identification software
Antemortem and postmortem records, photographs, x-rays ordered
Intact chain of evidence
All team members present or accounted for
Crime scene protocol completed or under completion
Preautopsy evidence collection is completed; the scene analysis is adequate
Defined course of action with time allocations made (for example, for lunch)
Environmental control intact; protective gear present
Evidence supplies and equipment double-checked for collection
Recording equipment is operative
Dissection tools are clean, sharp, and operative
Cell phones are off

Dirty Tricks at and with the Autopsy

Dirty tricks are not usually evil or malicious but attempts by other workers to get home early, skip out for a hot date, or make their day a little less tedious. Dirty tricks are stupid and sometimes misdirected hostility. They are always minor events.

Most dirty tricks are small and insignificant and not worthy of mention; they are not meant to harm. If you know that they exist, you can avoid most dirty tricks. Always respect yourself.

1. "We are out of blades (or towels, wipers, formalin, or some essential)."

   Response: Reach into your desk and pull out a backup. You have to keep backups for all essentials.

2. You arrive on time to find the autopsy room in a mess and uncleaned from the day before.

   Response: Change into your dissection clothes and do the mopping and cleaning quickly and start the autopsy as soon as you can.

3. "Your check has not come."

   Response: "Will it be here tomorrow?" Smile and await tomorrow.

4. You arrive on time for the autopsy but the police who will identify the body as that at the scene and provide the synopsis of the case are missing and their whereabouts unknown.

   Response: Use the time to be overprepared for the dissection. Take the time to clean and scrub your tools. Sharpen your tools and review/replenish your knife sharpening station. Replenish your stationery. Do some housekeeping duties at your desk. Wander over to talk with the secretaries who probably will tell you when the police will arrive.

5. You have a tox case to do and find out that the toxicology collection set and mailer is not to be found and the kit supply is gone.

   Response: Go to your file cabinet and pull out a backup kit. Include a note to the tox lab to quickly send you a replenishing supply of mail-off kits. Of course, you can scrounge up various clean tubes you have at your send-out station, make up (copy) your own form, provide a history, package the tubes securely with proper chain-of-evidence labeling and statements, call the tox lab and inform them what you are doing, and send it off (or take it to the lab yourself).

6. You come to the morgue and find an unidentified body in the cooler.

   Response: If you are the pathologist in charge of the morgue, then you have a big problem; if someone else is managing the morgue coolers it is less of a problem but still a problem. The body may need special attention (like prompt chemical analysis with immediate sample submission). This is the well-known problem of the unauthorized entry of a body to the morgue. It is usually a middle-of-the-night thing where someone with keys permits an undertaker to store a body overnight because of some personal problem, a funeral home mishap, or equivalent. This creates a sort of secondary scene event with the entire set of questions related to a scene now being played out at the morgue. You call the night man and talk. You talk with your police contact. You talk with all of the staff searching for an answer. Maybe the anthropologist or one of the psychiatric doctors will have an answer. You keep on the line until you make the right contact. Generally it is a do-gooder trying to help out a funeral director or a hospital. Occasionally it is a "country coroner" with no understanding of the protocol or etiquette.

7. You receive a subpoena in the mail for a civil proceeding or lawyer's office meeting on an old autopsy case without any antecedent communication.

   Response: Since there is no previous communication or meeting, since there is no pretrial communication here, and since you are not an officer of the court, you have no obligation to respond to this subpoena. The secretary can call. When you are the autopsy surgeon and not an elected governmental official (i.e., coroner or medical examiner), you have no responsibility or duty to unsolicited or unauthorized demands. A not-so-uncommon litigation procedure (which attempts to avoid any payment of a fee for pathologist cause-of-death testimony and avoid lawyer involvement in the blood-and-gore aspects of death cases) is to send notices that are known to be invalid and will not get a response. Of course, the lawyer has the privilege of arguing whatever aspects of an accident that he or she chooses; however, when both sides stipulate to the findings of the autopsy without any introspection, the ground is set for a limited analysis of the death and its circumstances. Many clerical workers have problems with cutting someone off and telling them that certain services are not provided by the medical staff. They want to be helpful to the caller. But it winds up as a call that you the professional has to turn down and refer when the clerks know the service is not provided.

8. You come to the morgue and find that there is a set of ceiling cameras installed and operative without any notice being given to you (the professional to be filmed and photographed) of their installation and how they will be used. Cameras and microphones may be installed in both open (you are notified) and closed (you are not notified) circumstances. The evidentiary circumstances of the visual and sound recordings need to be well understood by all involved who are recorded. The question is of course how far will the good will of employment be carried.

9. After your first autopsy of the day, you are asked about performing a second "outside" case. "Outside autopsies" are private autopsies conducted outside of the governmental or academic circumstances usually at the request of a private corporation, business, or legal firm to establish evidence favoring a solicited outcome. They may be primary or secondary (second time) autopsies and might support a known outcome.

Response: How you handle this situation is up to your terms of employment and the nature of the case. Be sure to clear it with management if you are not the management.

10. Often the police and prosecutors analyze our autopsy case results with a set end or purpose in mind. They have a story they want to validate. They may not start a case like the pathologist who has an open mind and an undetermined cause of death. For police and prosecutors, autopsy analysis is an undertaking that will favor or not favor an outcome they prefer.

The term "opinion shopping" may be applied to these circumstances. Of course, the desired method for opinion formation is to collect all of the available information and then evaluate the information independent of the personalities and circumstances involved. Opinion shopping is also used in interviewing the various physicians who have had contact with a homicide victim; the prosecution will highlight the viewpoints of the attendees, which provide a stronger offense statement. Generally witnesses do not speak of their cases with one another. However the attorney does have this capability and is able to fashion the medical testimony to fit his or her argument by omissions, duplications, blurring of observations, facts, and opinions, and other well known tricks of oral debate. Do not be surprised to find your time on the stand to be brief in some cases.

11. Talking on the cell phone while an autopsy is in progress: This is not a dirty trick; it is just bad manners. Someone in the autopsy viewing group gets a cell phone call while you are dissecting. They proceed have a lengthy conversation about their personal matters. How do you get respect for what you are doing? Or should we just accept disrespectful people? I usually just accept the bad manners excuse and carry on.

The Outside Expert Comes to Town: 10 Points

I use the news services of Yahoo and Google to cover forensic pathology, forensic pathologists, coroner, and medical examiner as topic areas. This daily service is free. I can download stories to my e-mail box and save them in a computer file.

After a few years of reading the entries, you find a rhythm and repetitive code to the stories that are covered. They concern job and personnel changes, special and routine cases, new operatives, and problems with jurisdiction. One well-covered topic is the work of outside experts who work all over the world, providing expert witness testimony. The outside expert is an important member of the medicolegal community and ensures a fair trial without the unregulated dominance of the state in scientific matters. Michael Baden, MD, and Cyril Wecht, MD, are well-regarded and experienced outside experts in matters of forensic science, pathology, and the autopsy. Many others are practicing forensic pathology solely as expert witnesses and list their practices in national and international directories. Some pathologists limit their courtroom appearances to the cases that belong to them through their autopsy skills. Thus, they defend their own findings. The outside expert has to bridge this gap and decide which way is the truth.

1. Not all experts are board certified by the American Board of Pathology. The curriculum vitae should be reviewed for appropriate educational qualifications. Errors in curriculum vitae are not unusual and can be very embarrassing.
2. Most are limited in their intelligence about the case by the limitations of the knowledge of the lawyer who hired them. If the lawyer is weak in the sciences, the materials reviewed may reflect this weakness and be incomplete.

3. Few pathologists do independent experimental research on their cases. This may be a major shortcoming in preparation. Since there are no limitations to those who commit murder in their wickedness, there are no limitations to those who attempt to discover their evil deeds. A forensic laboratory is always open to new technologies to discover the new methods of homicide that are perpetrated on the public each year. Independent experimental research is accepted in the forensic sciences.

4. Most experts will review the autopsy histological and cytological slides from the case when available. Then they become responsible for the accuracy of the previous diagnoses and for the accuracy of their own current diagnosis.

5. Specialist testimony may require the testimony of a subject interest specialist. These are found in the American Academy of Forensic Sciences and other organizations. Many such specialists have independent testimonial services; many are experienced engineers and technicians in the topic area.

6. Testifying experts may have marginal qualifications and approach the topic as with a pseudoscience. Some diseases are recognized which fail to provide any evidence of specificity or pathological distinction. Records of previous testimony are available to counter these problems. Expert testimony is not free of political viewpoint or attitude. Sometimes a goal of closing down a forensic functionary seems evident.

7. Testimony and expert testimony in particular, is not free. The going rate for an expert is $5,000 to start a contract. An outside autopsy has a pathologist fee of $3,000. Courtroom testimony is contracted by the number of days spent on the stand. The expenses of travel and accommodations are covered. Experts need malpractice insurance like everyone else, except those who are self-insured.

8. Pretrial preparation. Prepare, prepare, prepare. The witness must read all of the police, coroner, medical examiner, clinic, and hospital papers involved in the case. No inspection or examination can be left unreviewed. A theory for the trial must be agreed upon. A list of critical events and happenings in the case should be established and reviewed by the entire team. Preparation for the direct and cross-examination should be a first priority. A review of the medical aspects of the case can be made a separate but not independent task.

9. Surprises from witnesses. Witnesses may present some surprise answers if they are taken into unevaluated or untraveled territories. The witness must be protected from surprise questions so as not to give a confusing or obfuscating answer. The more experienced witnesses are slow and deliberate with good pronunciation and diction. Attention to detail should be the rule. Skill in oratorical rebuttal is an attribute. But not a necessity.

10. It takes some organization. The forensic witness when called cold on the telephone without preliminary notification is very liable to be negative to the caller. An anticipatory letter is gracious and most helpful. The scientific witness will need access to a scientific lab that meets his or her requirements for the review and evaluation of the items of the case and the facilities necessary to test any working hypotheses derived from the case and its evidence. In pathology, for instance, this would include access to an administrative team including a bookkeeper and tax consultant; a body transportation system including a private airplane and pilot; a body storage and autopsy area with radiological and imaging support; a full and complete histology, toxicology, informatics, and immunology laboratory with associated specialists capable of skilled testimony; an executive secretary; and media specialists.

Many testifying scientists use the facilities of their workplace to provide this core of specialization. And many get into problems with the bookkeeping of these operations. Even Russell S. Fisher MD, my mentor, had to defend his own Maryland Medicolegal Foundation from charges of corruption. Fisher started the foundation when the money from the Maryland race tracks proved insufficient to support the ancillary duties required for his office. These included entertaining new scientists and employees, help in moving staff, accommodations to visiting scientists, support of new technologies (e.g., ultrasound and photography), support of the required neuropathological services, and sending workers to meetings and conferences. He used the fees arising from the internal functioning of the office and fashioned them into his foundation. He put the fees for the training of various forensic specialists into the fund. Other fees and moneys derived from office products were placed in the foundation. He took the government moneys for training programs and put them into the foundation. The foundation became a successful monetary mechanism, had an independent board of directors, and was copied by organizations from all over the world. Fisher may historically be more significant in the development of the independent medicolegal foundation than in any of his other contributions.

The Minimal Activity Autopsy and Ten Cases a Day

In the large city and metropolitan morgues, the work of the coroner and medical examiner is a major undertaking of twenty-five or more cases a day. The pathologists work in groups of five, ten, fifteen, and twenty workers.

Sometimes even more. Work in this environment requires fast, accurate, and skillful dissection with a keen sense of attention to focal details. As an example, is the thrombotic focus in a smaller coronary or a septic brain lesion in a homeless schizophrenic.

The minimal activity autopsy is a complete opening of all of the body cavities with speed and accuracy. The scene sets the circumstances of suspicion; the initial view of the cavities sets the nature of the organ damage; and the dissection of the organs is focused on color, consistency, size, form, shape, and feel. The importance of consistency and feel is significant. Color is one of the last parameters of the autopsy that pathologists learn to appreciate and use. The gift of touch is limited by sanitary precautions and gloves. Any tailor or fabric user will speak to the importance of touch.

The minimal activity autopsy is a device so pathologists can examine many bodies in a limited time and yet provide a scientifically reliable death certificate. Commonly this autopsy form eliminates the running of the bowel, formalin fixation of the brain, extensive fluid collections for toxicology, complete histological review of normal appearing tissues, osteological descriptions, middle ear and sinus examinations, quantitative measurements of body fluids, skin cultures and biopsies, dental descriptions, fingerprinting, and proof of identity tests.

One caveat is necessary. When the fast autopsy on initial dissection fails to show a distinct and clear cause of death (e.g., fatty liver and/or pneumonia), the case analysis changes and the routine becomes the slow deliberate search for the cause of death.

Keeping Up with Medical Examiners and Coroners

I keep up with other medical examiners, coroners, forensic pathologists, and workers in the field of the forensic autopsy by having a daily selection of newspaper stories in the fields of forensic pathology, forensic autopsy, medical examiner, and coroner sent to me (free of charge) by the news services of Yahoo and Google. I print or save any interesting or unusual stories under a yearly file. I am able to follow the big-time forensic witnesses as they tour the world. I have over six years of selected forensic stories, and as you might suspect there is repetition over the years.

If you enter in specific names in Internet search engines, even more specific data is available. The professional utility of finding out the mistakes, errors, financial, and professional concerns of other forensic services is most valuable. The news services fulfill many of the social needs informatics of our profession.

The Incident Report and Quality Control

All quality control in the lab stems from the incident report. The incident report is a total listing of all defects in the lab service, lab environment, lab personnel capacities, and relationships. Once listed and made public, the event or item is ground through the administrative jungle and is recorded, defined, evaluated, discussed, given a remedy, correction, or at least a hearing. It is placed into a review system with doubling of administrative analysis and action. The corrective system is restated and a second calendar event is created and logged. The supervisors sign off with discussion; the chief signs off with a final evaluation. No event or happening is too small or unimportant.

Your Annual Report, Its Content, and Its Value

For those of us who work for themselves, the report to the Internal Revenue Service (IRS) or the moneylender is the annual report. However for the workers without ownership, the annual report is an essential item in their economic, business, and social relationships. Stop and make a lists of your accomplishments. Arrange them in some priority and cover all of your responsibilities. Defend your actions and explain your mistakes. Show a profit or show a loss; defend your financial status. Describe your accomplishments for the year. Tell of your fortunate experiences. Then explain your plans for the forthcoming year. Describe your goals. Anticipate events.

Present your report in several pages. Enumerate the major points for clearness. Distribute and file the report with those with whom you work and who would profit from its understanding. Personally compare it with your other reports.

Add your annual reports together and see if the direction of your work is where you want it.

It's Not Your Business: Working for Others, the Government, and Universities; Your Social Consciousness

On reviewing your finances and your income structure as a pathologist, do not forget that most pathologists finish their training with family expenses and without sufficient capital to go out and start a lab of their own. Although some business advisers will tout you to always work for someone else and have them take care of the business details, there are times in pathology where independence from another professional's overview allows for some worthwhile independent and original thinking. As a professional you will ponder this employment dilemma on and off your entire career. Think it over, but remember it will recur and reinvent itself time and time again. However, it looks like scientific medical practice is getting more remote economically from the ordinary medical pathologist entrepreneur.

Stewardship is an important concept for any professional. It means that you take responsibility not only for the job that you do, but that also you take responsibility for all of the parts of your social assignment whether you are actively involved with them or not. This is your social responsibility and derives from your social consciousness. The stewardship of the forensic pathologist is not only for his own autopsy service but for the entire autopsy service for the community that he serves. As physicians we abide by the Hippocratic oath and work for perfection in the provision of medical services. A professional does not have to be reminded of the stewardship of his profession. He or she has a social consciousness.

What Is a "Hot Shop?"

I first heard this expression from Charles Petty, MD, when working with him at the Baltimore office. As with any human service activity in which there is an aggregation of learned and experienced personnel, there are times when aggregates of people form exceptional groups that extend the capacities of the usual service group. These exceptional groupings of skilled and intelligent artisans are called "hot shops." A hot shop is an organization that is leading the way into the future by understanding and using new technologies and theories in a formidable fashion. Some medical examiner and coroner offices may push forward the science of forensic pathology and allow new procedures, new laws, new instruments, new software, new ethics, and new advances to be made that affect their practice and that of others practicing. Such a group may produce an atlas, a book, a new instrument, a new disease description, a new disease vector, a new drug or chemical, or maybe an entirely different method of correcting social evils. All forensic scientists interested in learning are on the lookout for hot shops—either to imitate, join, visit, evaluate, emulate, or photograph.

Charles Petty MD

Charles Petty was one of the most influential pathologists and forensic scientists in America during the second half of the twentieth century. He would want to be remembered as first of all a true gentleman who was always concerned with the welfare of his students and his co-workers while maintaining the dignity of the profession of forensic pathology. He fostered by his example active participation of pathologists in organized medicine. He served as the president of American Academy of Forensic Sciences in the 1960s. The

British forensic sciences were a subject of his study. He studied at Harvard and was a candidate for the chair there when unfortunately the pivotal 1966 mistake of dropping the Harvard School of Legal Medicine was made, a blow which a half century later has still not been rectified. Charles went on to lead the Baltimore, Indiana, and Dallas offices into national forces in forensic pathology. As a forensic scientist, he promoted definitive case solution with strong analytical, toxicological, and anatomical pathology evidence with forensic science support as available. He was concerned with the proper presentation of forensic evidence in the courtroom. He worked many trials with pride and accomplishment. He had many friends wherever he went, his students especially. He certainly knew the history and national evolution of forensic pathology.

Looking back, I note he was not big into writing for grants. He was more concerned with his efforts in presenting his cases properly in the courts. Maybe this is true for many other forensic scientists of that age. Undoubtedly it is conditioned by the lack of research funding by the federal government into things forensic. Of course, the FBI was a big player in this game and probably needed all of the funding they could get.

The Role of the Relational Database to Scientific Forensics

You studied Excel and know how to arrange a worksheet with your data and call it a datasheet. Now to arrange the data and sort it out with different relationships of the data you will need to create relationships between the items in your datasheets. You need to learn how to work relational databases. You need to program your relational database.

Like everything else in computers, there are big relational database programs and little relational databases. Microsoft Access is the relational database program for general consumption, requires no licensing of its users, is part of the Microsoft Office program set, is the cheapest package yet very powerful and expandable. This is the one I use. I do not use the larger relational databases QST or Oracle. These programs are more expensive (although student editions are available) and require licensing of the relational database operation. For single operative scientists, I recommend Access. For large metropolitan offices, you can use Access, Oracle, or QST. Regardless, the dynamics of computer management of a relational database is not for children and requires study and repetition.

All systems are based on the analytical power of the list. The list being the grouping of similar objects and things that can be compared to one another. The list makes the table, the table makes the form for reporting and record keeping. The table makes the query to compare items from lists to one another. The query makes the report that arranges the list data in proper form. The essentials of relational databases are found in these words: list, table, form, query, report, project.

Conclusion

In my practice over the years, certain experiences stand out and might be of interest to those who follow. While I practice to solve practical problems (pathology cases), my individuality is projected in my scientific endeavors, which are explanations and descriptions of the natural phenomenon I have encountered and described. Becoming a scientist is a separate mission from becoming a practitioner of medicine. In my circumstances of searching for admission to medical school, becoming a practicing scientist was a second major benefit. I have learned to use and appreciate that experience in a positive manner and am thankful for it.

Dedication

IV

Dedication to
Russell S. Fisher, MD

It is fitting to revise the forensic pathology objectives and more fitting to dedicate this work to my formal mentor in forensic pathology, Russell S. Fisher, MD. Fisher gave me an open door when Harvard closed theirs; Fisher gave me and hundreds of others their real key to the science of forensic pathology. He collaborated with his alma mater, Harvard, and the New York, Philadelphia, Washington DC, and Virginia offices. He worked this country for forensic pathology. He built the Maryland office into a national resource for training and service expertise. Fisher worked hard to promote the role of the forensic consultant in trial law by his travels, teachings, and labors. Fisher promoted the training of pathologists in forensic pathology by consulting and advising tens of programs in the westward expansion of forensic pathology in the 1950s through 1970s. He promoted the broad expanse of forensic pathology, mentored independent research affiliates to major offices, led forensic pathology into prominence in the American Academy of Forensic Sciences, and started the utilization of the federal research grant funds into support of forensic research. He was a champion of research in crib deaths with several of his students becoming prominent leaders in SIDS work. Fisher helped to establish neuropathology as an integral part of forensic pathology practice and an essential skill area for individual forensic pathologists. All forensic pathologists should honor his bibliography and his life. He was a selfless champion of forensic pathology.

His writings as the chief medical examiner of the State of Maryland during the 1950s and 1960s are available on the Web site of the National Library of Medicine (www.pubmed.gov). It includes the following articles written by and about Fisher

1. Fisher, R. S., Katz, S. S., and Lovitt, W. V. Sudden Deaths in Infancy. A Sociopathological Study. Report from the Office of the Chief Medical Examiner of Maryland and Department of Legal Medicine. Baltimore: University of Maryland Medical School, 1959.
2. Corrigan, G. E., and Fisher, R. S. Sudden unexpected death in infants. *Maryland State Medical Journal* 18 (1969): 70–72.
3. Spitz, W. V., and Fisher, R. S., eds. *Medicolegal Investigation of Death*, 2nd ed. Springfield, IL: C.C. Thomas, 1974.

4. Fisher's papers on boric acid lethality to suckling infants were important in highlighting pediatric toxicological problems. Some mothers were using boric acid powder to treat their babies' skin problems and deaths were discovered due to boric acid poisoning. It was quickly taken off the market for use in pediatric care.

5. Correspondence and lectures on the utility of a medical examiner's private foundation for research, improvement, and growth were critical in the growth and expansion of pathology.

6. Taylor, B. The case of the outspoken medical examiner or an exclusive interview with Russell S. Fisher, MD, chief medical examiner of the state of Maryland. *Maryland State Medical Journal* 26, no. 3 (1977): 59–61, 63–70.

7. Petty, C. S. The medical examiner and medical education (Russell S. Fisher). *Human Pathology* 11, no. 2 (1980): 101–103.

8. Spitz, W. U. A tribute to the late Russell S. Fisher. *American Journal of Forensic Medical Pathology* 9, no. 4 (1988): 355–356.

Index

For Product Safety Concerns and Information please contact our EU
representative GPSR@taylorandfrancis.com
Taylor & Francis Verlag GmbH, Kaufingerstraße 24, 80331 München, Germany